ALZHEIMER'S
DISEASE
THE COMPLETE
INTRODUCTION

Works on Alzheimer's by the Same Authors

Poirier, Judes, ed. "Apoptosis: Techniques and Protocols."
Neuromethods 29. New York: Humana Press, 1997.

Gauthier, S., A. Burns, and W. Petit. *Alzheimer's Disease in
Primary Care*. London: Martin Dunitz, 1997.

Gauthier, S., A. Burns, and W. Petit. *La Maladie d'Alzheimer
en Médecine Générale*. London: Martin Dunitz, 1997.

Gauthier, S., ed. *Pharmacotherapy of Alzheimer's Disease*.
London: Martin Dunitz, 1998.

Gauthier, S., ed. *Clinical Diagnosis and Management of Alzheimer's
Disease*. Rev. 2nd ed. London: Martin Dunitz, 2001.

Erkinjutti, T. and S. Gauthier, ed. *Vascular Cognitive Impairment*.
London: Martin Dunitz, 2002.

Gauthier, S., P. Scheltens, and J. Cummings, ed. *Alzheimer's Disease and
Related Disorders*. London: Martin Dunitz/Taylor & Francis, 2005.

Gauthier S., ed. *Clinical Diagnosis and Management of Alzheimer's Disease*.
3rd ed. London: Informa Healthcare, 2007.

Wahlund, L.O., T. Erkinjutti, and S. Gauthier, ed. *Vascular Cognitive Impairment
in Clinical Practice*. Cambridge: Cambridge University Press, 2009.

Gauthier, S. and C. Ballard. *Management of Dementia*. London:
Informa Healthcare, 2009.

Dr. Judes Poirier
Dr. Serge Gauthier

ALZHEIMER'S
DISEASE
THE COMPLETE
INTRODUCTION

Translated by Barbara Sandilands

Foreword by André Chagnon

Afterword by the Right Honourable
Michaëlle Jean

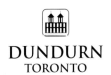

DUNDURN
TORONTO

Editor: Michael Melgaard
Design: Courtney Horner
Printer: Transcontinental

Library and Archives Canada Cataloguing in Publication

Poirier, Judes, 1961-
[Maladie d'Alzheimer. English]
Alzheimer's disease : the complete introduction / Dr. Judes Poirier & Dr.
Serge Gauthier ; foreword by André Chagnon ; afterword by Michaëlle Jean
; translated by Barbara Sandilands.

Translation of: La maladie d'Alzheimer.
Includes bibliographical references.
Issued in print and electronic formats.
ISBN 978-1-4597-2350-4

1. Alzheimer's disease. I. Gauthier, Serge, 1950-, author II. Sandilands,
Barbara, translator III. Title. IV. Title: Maladie d'Alzheimer. English.

RC523.P6513 2014   616.8'31   C2013-908380-4
                                                          C2013-908381-2

        1   2   3   4   5   18   17   16   15   14

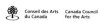 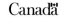 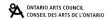

We acknowledge the support of the **Canada Council for the Arts** and the **Ontario Arts Council** for our publishing
program. We also acknowledge the financial support of the **Government of Canada** through the **Canada Book Fund**
and **Livres Canada Books**, and the **Government of Ontario** through the **Ontario Book Publishing Tax Credit** and the
Ontario Media Development Corporation.

Care has been taken to trace the ownership of copyright material used in this book. The author and the publisher welcome
any information enabling them to rectify any references or credits in subsequent editions.
J. Kirk Howard, President

The publisher is not responsible for websites or their content unless they are owned by the publisher.

Printed and bound in Canada.

Visit us at
Dundurn.com | @dundurnpress | Facebook.com/dundurnpress | Pinterest.com/Dundurnpress

Dundurn	Gazelle Book Services Limited	Dundurn
3 Church Street, Suite 500	White Cross Mills	2250 Military Road
Toronto, Ontario, Canada	High Town, Lancaster, England	Tonawanda, NY
M5E 1M2	LA1 4XS	U.S.A. 14150

This book is dedicated to Francine, Louise, Thérèse, Éric, Judith, Catherine, and Alexandre for having helped us stay the course through the ups and downs of life.

Table of Contents

Foreword

If there is one subject that has been constantly on my mind for several years, it's Alzheimer's disease, for my wife, Lucie, is suffering from it. Like many families, we are coping with the situation and learning to mourn the loss of a number of pleasures that only death should have taken away. Communication, closeness, and shared dreams are no longer possible. Of course, Lucie is not the only person with this disease. There are forty million victims worldwide, and that number is expected to reach eighty million in the space of a generation.

Alzheimer's disease is beginning to take on epidemic proportions and will severely affect Canadians, given our aging population. To paraphrase Jean de La Fontaine, the famous writer of fables, it's safe to say that while not everyone will personally fall victim to the disease, we will all be affected by it. Without question, each of us will see members of our family or immediate circle diagnosed and in need of care.

On a daily basis, caregivers need encouragement, support, and advice to help them fulfill their role and make good decisions. As for the upcoming generation, they need to know whether research is progressing and whether they can hope for a less worrying future than that of their parents and grandparents. This book provides answers to both questions in clear and easily understood terms. It offers advice to caregivers and dispels myths by providing accurate data and medical explanations to help younger readers understand.

Well-known for their expertise in this field, Drs. Judes Poirier and Serge Gauthier have successfully taken stock of both past and current research, even making a brief foray into the future. Their approach to the aspects of the disease is straightforward and rigorous. Genetics, risk factors, making a diagnosis, the progression of the disease, treatments, prevention — it's all here. We are very lucky that many researchers and clinicians are devoting so much energy to advancing research in this field, and the information provided by the authors offers a kind of comforting reassurance.

If I could have one wish, it would be for the book *Alzheimer's Disease: The Complete Introduction* to find its way into people's homes even before the onset of symptoms. There is a very simple reason for this: it is much easier to deal with the subject in a family when no one has the disease. A person who waits until he suspects his spouse is showing signs of the disease before reading this book may be running the risk of eliciting an angry reaction when the spouse sees what he has been reading. All needless conflict situations involving a person with Alzheimer's disease must be avoided, in favour of an understanding, respectful, and loving approach. We have to realize that the vast majority of people in the initial phase of the disease tend to deny they have symptoms and refuse even to discuss them.

No one can claim that preventive measures are effective in every case, but they certainly can't hurt. A healthy diet, physical exercise, and education, among others, will always guarantee a better quality of life, and they must be encouraged. Although the mission of the Lucie and André Chagnon foundation is not to prevent Alzheimer's disease, prevention is at the heart of everything the foundation does. In every field, I believe that prevention should be the priority; this is even more the case with respect to research on Alzheimer's disease, for the human and financial costs for our society are going to increase dramatically in the coming years.

Treatments have progressed a great deal since the disease was identified a hundred years ago, and doctors have more sophisticated ways of attending to patients. I have the opportunity to observe this every day I see Dr. Gauthier, who has been looking after my wife since 2004. Through his humane approach, he has succeeded in creating a close bond over the years, both with Lucie and with our family, for which I am profoundly grateful.

ANDRÉ CHAGNON
CHAIRMAN AND CHIEF EXECUTIVE OFFICER
LUCIE AND ANDRÉ CHAGNON FOUNDATION

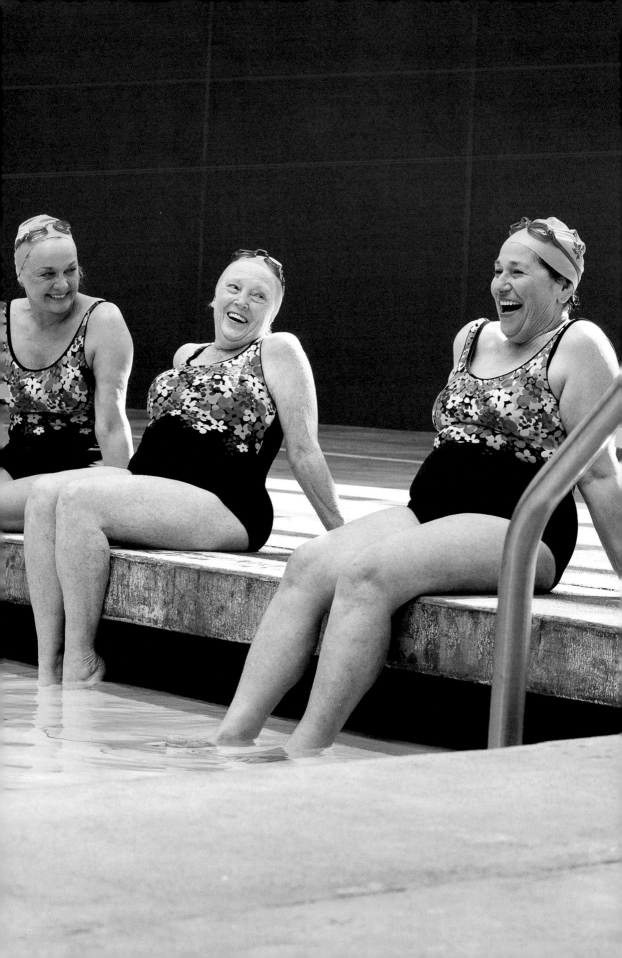

Alzheimer's Disease in the Baby Boomer Era

The medical profession has, for many years, tended to associate gradual memory loss with normal aging. Hence the surprising statistic that more than 50 percent of people with mild Alzheimer's disease are not diagnosed, or are diagnosed but not treated. It is important to realize that, for a long time, the large family of dementias to which Alzheimer's disease belongs, was of little or no interest to doctors, as its main symptoms were considered to be the natural consequences of aging.

Not everyone deemed Alzheimer's to be a disease in the true sense of the word — one with a predictable clinical progression and measurable symptoms. It was instead seen as the consequence of growing older. Often, the initial symptoms have only a very small impact on a person's day-to-day activities. It is thus quite rare to see individuals in the mild stage go by themselves to the doctor to discuss their symptoms. Usually someone close to the person (the spouse or a relative) convinces the person that he or she needs to have a doctor assess the situation. In the affected person's mind everything seems fine and there is no need to see a doctor.

Figure 1 illustrates the progression of the major symptoms of Alzheimer's disease. As can be seen, the first phase, in which brain damage occurs very slowly over one or two decades, is silent, with no visible symptoms. When the first symptoms (such as a decline in short-term memory or the need to search for words) appear, the disease can be diagnosed. It is not uncommon at this stage for the patient or family to postpone seeing a doctor due to the belief that memory loss is completely normal in people of a certain age.

It has been observed that memory disorders tend to be predominant at the outset of the disease and become worse during the early years. Then follows a gradual loss of functional independence — the ability to manage one's finances, drive a car, prepare meals, and, eventually, take care of oneself and attend to one's basic needs. Later, behavioural problems quite often appear, varying both from one individual to another and by gender. Specifically, these include spontaneous outbursts of anger, aggressiveness, or, conversely, apathy and lack of interest. In the later stages, motor problems develop in a large portion of people affected, depriving them of their physical independence.

As can be seen, Alzheimer's is much more than a disease of the memory. It develops slowly in those sixty-five and older and affects regions of the brain where memory, learning, judgement, emotions, and even movement are controlled. And the fact is that the first baby boomers, the vanguard of the anticipated wave of aging adults who were born after World War II, have just turned sixty-five. The disease is expected to become more and more prevalent in the coming years.

This book offers a detailed analysis of the current state of the disease, its progression over time, and the efforts being made by various medical bodies to slow its progression or effectively manage some of its most problematic symptoms. Above all, the book tries to demystify the disease as a whole and to answer the most common questions asked by patients or members of their family. It presents a systematic review of more than a hundred years of medical research, including both the promising and not-so-promising results. It offers a regional and global view of Alzheimer's disease today and the choices our society will have to face in the relatively near future.

This book provides an overview of the latest medical and scientific news about

PROGRESSION OF ALZHEIMER'S DISEASE

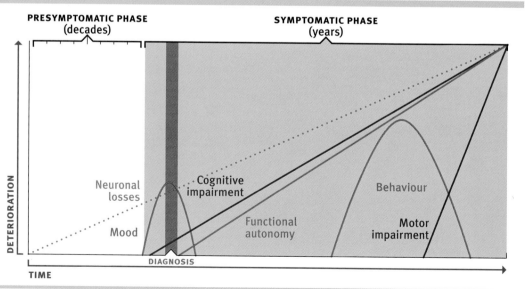

FIGURE 1

recent progress in research, the causes of and treatments for Alzheimer's disease, approaches to prevention that are being developed, and lifestyle habits that have been scientifically validated and may slow down or hinder the symptomatic progression of the disease. Among the many factors discussed are diet and exercise, two personal choices requiring neither a visit to the doctor nor a prescription.

Recent demographic data collected by various Alzheimer's societies around the world paint a rather dismal picture of the next three decades: ever more people affected, astronomical health-care costs, treatments that appear to have only limited effects, and half-hearted investment in research. Knowing this, we felt it was all the more important to explain the situation more fully to readers, to dispel certain myths that persist even today, and to describe, in a more humane way, the various stages of the disease and the choices a family must make at each step of the way. In short, we felt we had to tell it like it is, without being alarmist or getting caught up in hollow debates.

The medical community understands the disease much better than it did five years ago. We have gone from the stage where detecting the disease was difficult to developing sophisticated prevention strategies. It is this new understanding of causes and treatments that we want to share with readers in a non-technical, easily accessible way.

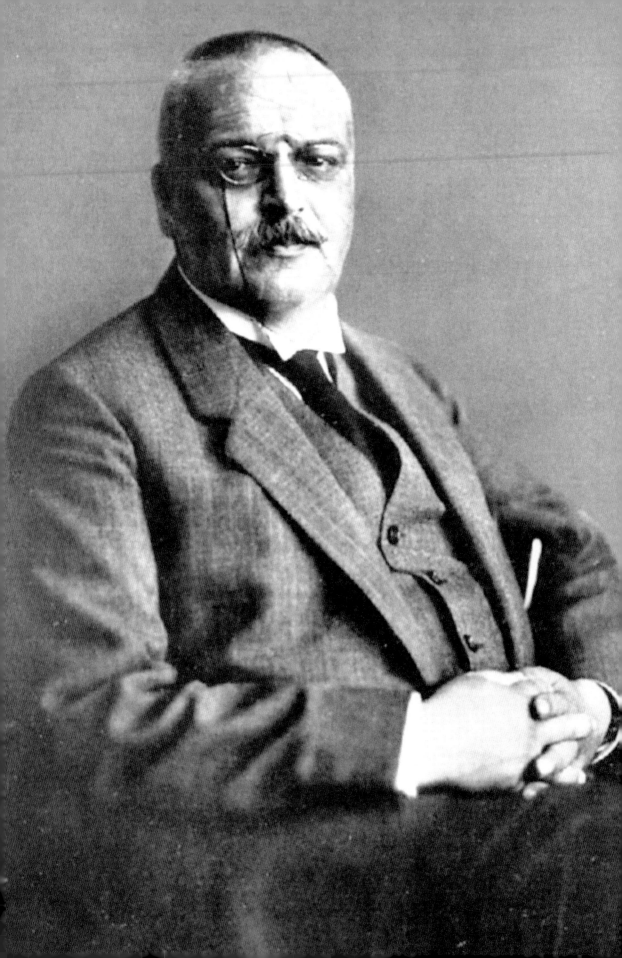

CHAPTER 1

Professor Alois Alzheimer: A Scientist with Heart

Born on June 14, 1864, in the small Bavarian town of Marktbreit, in Germany, Aloysius or Alois Alzheimer was the second son of royal notary Eduard Alzheimer. His birth went smoothly and he was baptized two weeks later, according to the Catholic rite of the time, in his father's house. Restored in 1995 by the Eli Lilly pharmaceutical company, the house has since been turned into a museum and a renowned international conference centre.

Little Alois had a carefree childhood. He attended his neighbourhood school until 1874, the year his father decided to send him to live with his uncle in Aschaffenburg, where he would continue his studies at that town's school. After Alois's birth, five other brothers and sisters were born into the family. Needing more space, the whole family eventually decided to join his father's older brother in Aschaffenburg.

In 1883 Alois graduated from high school. His professors noted in their written report: "This candidate has demonstrated exceptional knowledge in the natural sciences, which he showed a particular preference for during his years at school." He lost his mother shortly before finishing high school. His father later remarried and had one more child.

Concern for their fellow human beings was a tradition in the Alzheimer family and led several members to go into teaching or the priesthood. Alois saw an opportunity in the medical profession to combine his personal interests in the natural sciences and human relations, a passion that drove his life until his death at fifty-one. Although his older brother had suggested he join him in the university city of Würzburg, Alois decided to undertake his university medical studies in Berlin.

↖ Professor Alois Alzheimer, circa 1910.

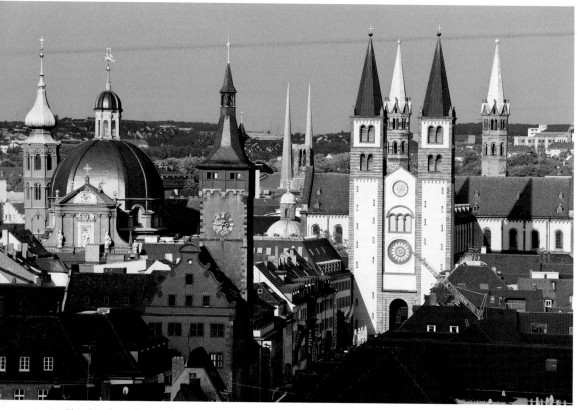

↖ The city of Würzburg today.

He officially entered the Faculty of Medicine at Royal Friedrich Wilhelm University in the autumn of 1883. Professor Waldeyer's anatomy courses fascinated him. The renowned pathologist had published a ground-breaking scientific article on the development of cancer, an article that challenged the established dogmas of the day. Interestingly, this work still forms the basis of several different avenues of research examining the spread of cancers in the human body. Alzheimer continued his studies the following year in the city of Würzburg, where he felt closer to home. There he discovered fencing, a sport he played with great enthusiasm until the day he received a fairly serious facial wound that left him with a deep scar — this wound was

the reason Alzheimer nearly always refused to be photographed from the right side.

In the winter of 1886, Alzheimer left the University of Würzburg to do a more advanced internship at the University of Tübingen. As a young man, his considerable height (1.8 metres) gave him a physically powerful look and earned him a certain degree of respect from the other students. Some twenty years later, Alzheimer would return to this very university to give an intriguing and historical lecture on a "new disease of the cerebral cortex" at a German medical conference.

Finally, in May 1888, Alzheimer passed the examinations of the Würzburg Medical Examination Board with first-class honours. That same year, Sigmund Freud presented the rudiments of what would later become psychoanalysis, a new branch of medicine arguing for the novel concept of healing through words. Meanwhile, Alzheimer introduced the use of the microscope in psychiatry, but frequently insisted on having private conversations with his patients. It was at this time that he began seriously asking questions about the biological roots of so-called "mental" illnesses.

In the period when Alzheimer was beginning his career as a physician and psychiatrist, two entirely different philosophies were at odds with each other to explain the origin of mental illnesses. Members of the first group, known as "psychists," were convinced that these illnesses were purely psychological in origin and could therefore be treated only by manipulating thoughts.

The "somatics," on the other hand, believed that disorders affecting the mentally ill were organic or biological in origin. These two diametrically opposed views often came into conflict at scientific or medical gatherings. Thus, physicians like Alzheimer, who were interested in biological and pathological changes in their patients, were generally poorly regarded among "psychists" like Freud.

It was in this very particular context that young doctor Alois Alzheimer, then twenty-four, left Würzburg to join the medical team at the Frankfurt am Main psychiatric hospital (Verhey, 2009). Called the "lunatics' castle" by the local population, this psychiatric hospital was one of the largest complexes of its kind in Germany. Built in gothic style, and without the traditional high walls of psychiatric institutions of the period, it stood outside the city of Frankfurt. A year later, a young doctor named Franz Nissl joined Alzheimer's team. There was a desperate lack of staff in the huge complex, which usually only accepted the most serious cases of mental illness. Today, Nissl is recognized as one of the pioneers in cerebral microscopy and one of the most enthusiastic defenders of the theory that mental illnesses are biological in origin. The two young doctors, under the kindly authority of Dr. Emil Sioli, undertook to completely change the way care was provided to

COMPARISON OF BEHAVIOURAL THEORIES IN THE EARLY TWENTIETH CENTURY

Psychic in origin (psychological)	Somatic in origin (biological)
Difficulties concentrating	Heart beats faster
Worries too much	Hands tremble
Has terrible hallucinations	Has diarrhea
Is anxious	Has a knot in the stomach
Has overwhelming thoughts	Walks back and forth
Is terrified	Feels listless

FIGURE 2

Professor Sigmund Freud, 1922.

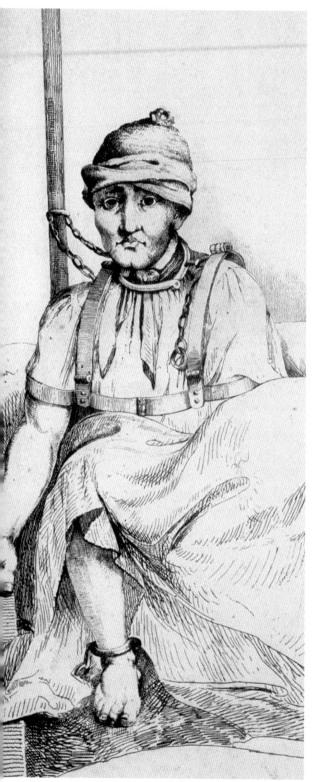

patients by putting into practice the so-called "no-constraints" approach (Engstrom, 2007). The coercive methods then in use were gradually dropped, replaced by greater and more responsible freedom of movement.

In the following years, Alzheimer first took an interest in psychoses that were biological in origin, often resulting in the active degeneration of blood vessels or the brain. Later, when he applied his scientific research in Munich, he became interested in "endogenous" psychoses, such as schizophrenia, manic depression, and the group of what are known as "early-onset" dementias. Thanks to his friend and colleague Nissl, who taught him cerebral histopathology techniques, Alzheimer was quick to make a link between the symptoms of patients he saw on a daily basis and microscopic analyses of the brains of patients who had died of these same illnesses.

THE CASE OF AUGUSTE DETER

Despite his departure from Frankfurt for Munich in 1903, Alzheimer had not forgotten the strange patient he had met for the first time in November 1901 (Verhey, 2009). At the time, Alzheimer was head physician at Frankfurt's psychiatric hospital. His assistant, Dr. Nitsch, had examined a new fifty-one-year-old patient on her arrival at the hospital. He had decided to talk about her specific case with his supervisor, suspecting a very odd abnormality. Alzheimer had agreed to go and see the patient, a meeting that would completely change the direction of the rest of his career.

↖ A patient incarcerated in the Bethlem Royal Psychiatric Hospital, known as Bedlam, in London, c. 1800.

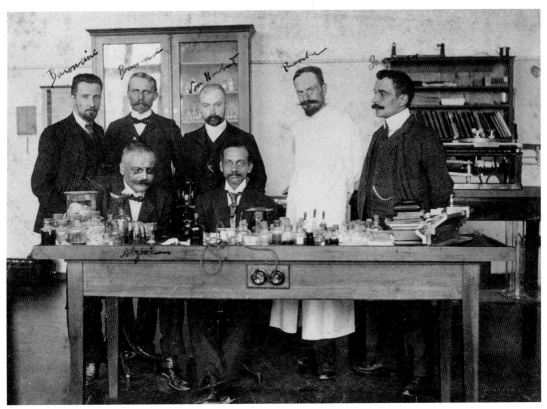

↗ A group of psychiatrists, including Professor Alzheimer (seated on the left), in the University of Munich hospital, c. 1905.

Right from their first conversations, Alzheimer became deeply fascinated by the patient, whose mood shifted constantly back and forth between gloom and contentment. She remembered her name very well, but had forgotten what year she was born. She was fully aware that she had a daughter living very nearby who had been married several years earlier in Berlin.

However, when Alzheimer asked her what her husband's name was, she could not remember. Nor did she know what hospital she was in or how long she had been there. On this surprising note Alzheimer's investigations began; he had already seen a few patients with similar traits, although none displaying so many inconsistencies all at once (Maurer et al., 1997). A general examination indicated this was a person in good health. A neurological examination appeared normal, aside from a few minor abnormalities. Periods of lucidity quickly gave way to incoherent and sometimes even aggressive behaviour. The patient frequently appeared anxious and sometimes very distrustful.

Auguste Deter's case fascinated Dr. Alzheimer. He remembered having observed, in previous years, cases of dementia that he had referred to at the time as cases of senility, since the subjects were much older than Auguste Deter, who was in her very early fifties. In 1885, the examination of one of these patients had revealed a significant loss of neuronal cells in the brain and lymph glands, even when

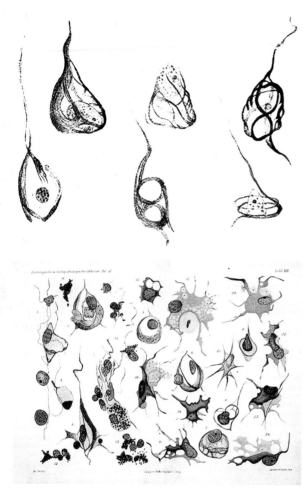

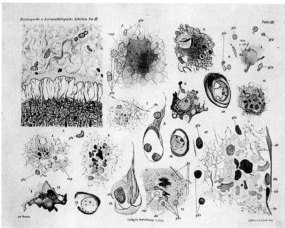

↖ Neurofibrillary tangles from Auguste Deter's brain drawn by Professor Alzheimer (top and centre); plaques from Auguste Deter's brain (bottom).

there was absolutely no blockage of the cerebral blood vessels. The doctor's notes show that he suspected a hereditary weakness of the central nervous system to be at the root of the decrease in brain cells.

Auguste Deter's husband had told the doctors that she had always enjoyed very good health and had never had any serious infectious diseases. She did not drink and he felt she was very hard-working. He had stressed that until 1901 his wife had never shown any particular symptoms. Then suddenly, that autumn, she had begun to experience memory lapses and frequently lied to cover up some of her "absences" (Maurer et al., 1997). A few weeks later, she began to have trouble preparing meals and had sometimes begun to wander aimlessly around the apartment. Shortly before being hospitalized, she had started to hide all kinds of objects, plunging the apartment into a state of chaos that did not make any sense at all to her husband.

The preferred treatment prescribed by Alzheimer at the time consisted of taking lukewarm baths. He received encouraging results by recommending a rest in the afternoon and a light meal in the evening. Tea and coffee were forbidden. Sleeping pills were only administered when absolutely necessary. But, a year after being hospitalized, Auguste Deter became constantly agitated and very anxious. At night, she frequently got out of bed and disturbed the other patients. Communication with the patient became extremely difficult and not very productive. In the final note on the file written by Alzheimer himself, he noted that the patient had become violent when he tried to listen to her chest. She cried for no reason and had almost stopped eating.

The stages of the disease as they are described here by Dr. Alzheimer are fairly typical of the normal progression of subjects with the disease that today bears his name. In his day, managing the patient's symptoms was difficult, not to say primitive, from some points of view. Fortunately, the situation has changed greatly since then. The variety of treatments available to people with the disease today make possible better management of the symptoms, as well as the behavioural problems that arise later on in the course of the disease. We will discuss treatment again in greater detail in later chapters of this book.

In April 1906, in Frankfurt, Alzheimer learned of Auguste Deter's death. He immediately asked his former mentor, Dr. Emil Sioli, to send him the patient's medical file and, if possible, her brain.

The director agreed. Reviewing the patient's file, Alzheimer discovered she had died from a serious case of pneumonia. Her illness (the one being examined) had lasted almost five years. Professor Alzheimer then got to work and prepared the late Auguste Deter's brain for a thorough microscopic analysis of its various regions.

He found noticeable atrophy of the cerebral lobes, a pronounced loss of neuronal cells in several sub-regions of the brain, and the presence of strange fibrillary pathology inside the neuronal cells. He also reported the existence of enormous fibrous glial cells (or feeder cells) and many biological deposits resembling spherical plaques (commonly known as senile plaques) throughout the patient's brain, as well as in the brain's blood vessels (Goedert and Ghetti, 2007). The sum total of all of these changes reminded Alzheimer and his

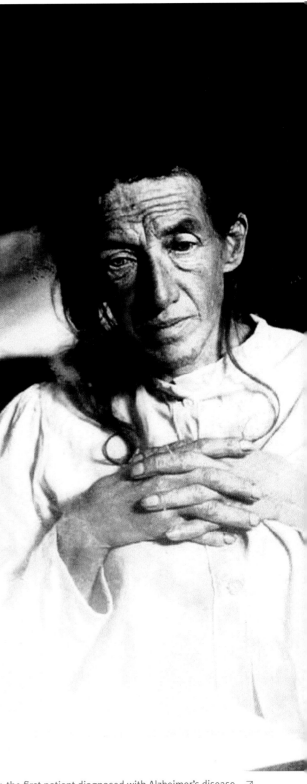

Auguste Deter, the first patient diagnosed with Alzheimer's disease. ↗

23

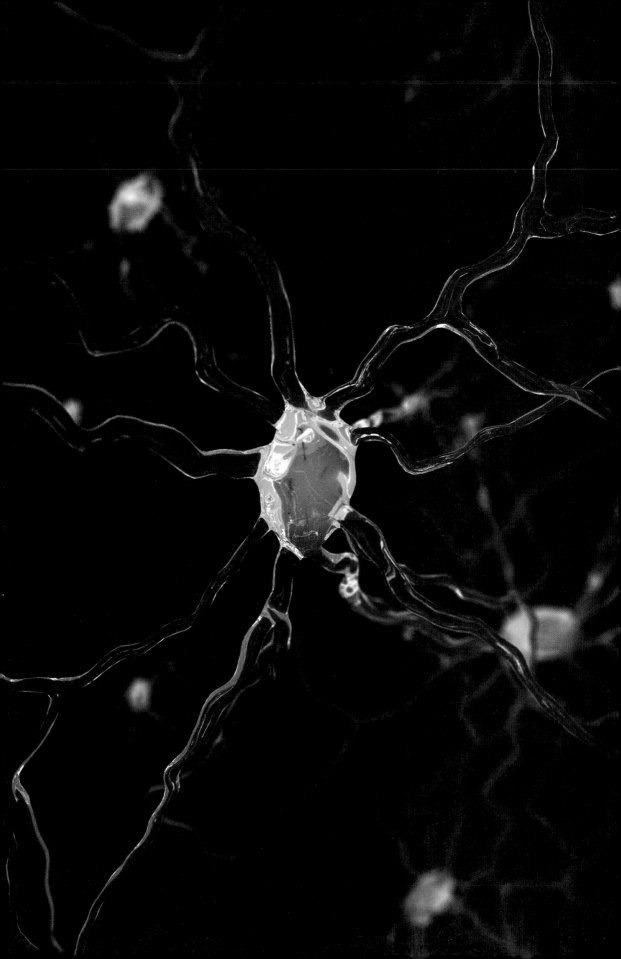

colleagues of the pathological characteristics of another illness, *Dementia senilis* (or senile dementia), commonly seen in very elderly people.

Thus, with solid support from rigorous clinical and pathological observations, Alzheimer arrived at the Thirty-seventh Conference of South-West German psychiatrists on November 3, 1906, to present the case of Auguste D. to the German scientific community. Once Alzheimer's presentation was over, the chair of the session opened up a question period. Surprisingly, Alzheimer was not asked a single question about his presentation or his patient. He left the Tübingen conference disappointed.

A year later, however, the situation was quite the opposite. Three patients suffering from the same disease arrived at the hospital during the year. Clinical and biological analyses of the three new cases confirmed the accuracy of Alzheimer's earlier work on Auguste Deter's illness

(Maurer et al., 1997). There really was a progressive neurodegenerative disease that damaged brain tissues and caused the pathological markers described earlier to appear, followed by the symptoms so typical of the disease. Yet it was not until 1909 that the pathological and clinical details of the four patients were formally published in a German medical journal, and it was 1910 before it was first referred to as "Alzheimer's disease."

His scientific renown spread beyond the borders of Germany and his work earned him international fame. Since the concept of "Alzheimer's disease" had been identified during his lifetime, he was able to enjoy the recognition of his peers despite the initial lack of interest shown by the doctors who had attended his scientific presentation in 1906. Alois Alzheimer died in Breslau on December 19, 1915, at the age of fifty-two, after a long kidney illness.

TRANSVERSAL SECTION OF THE BRAIN SHOWING NEURONAL CELLS

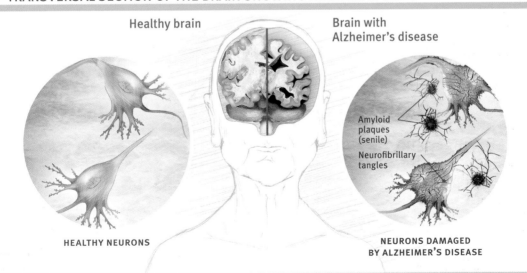

Healthy brain

Brain with Alzheimer's disease

Amyloid plaques (senile)

Neurofibrillary tangles

HEALTHY NEURONS

NEURONS DAMAGED BY ALZHEIMER'S DISEASE

FIGURE 3

◤ A model of neurons connected by synapses.

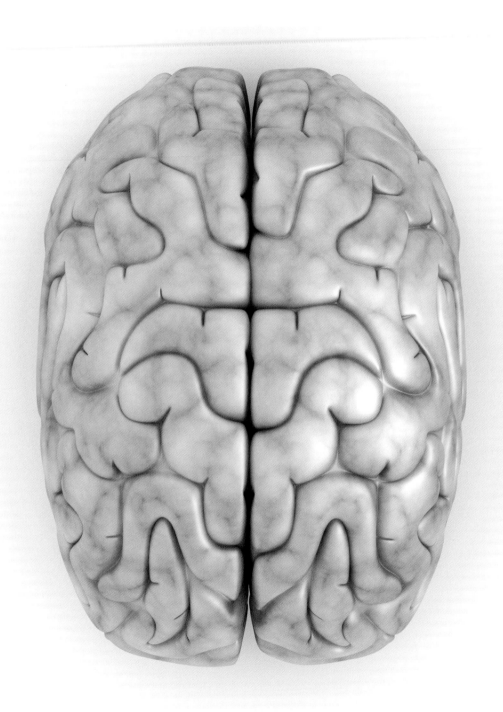

In Summary

Professor Alois Alzheimer: A Scientist With Heart

A German psychiatrist born in Marktbreit in 1864, Alois Alzheimer observed in 1901 the symptoms of a new disease in a patient named Auguste Deter, who died in 1906. This disease, which would come to bear his name, was described in scientific literature for the first time in 1910. Its characteristics include serious memory disorders, a progressive deterioration in judgement, and behavioural problems.

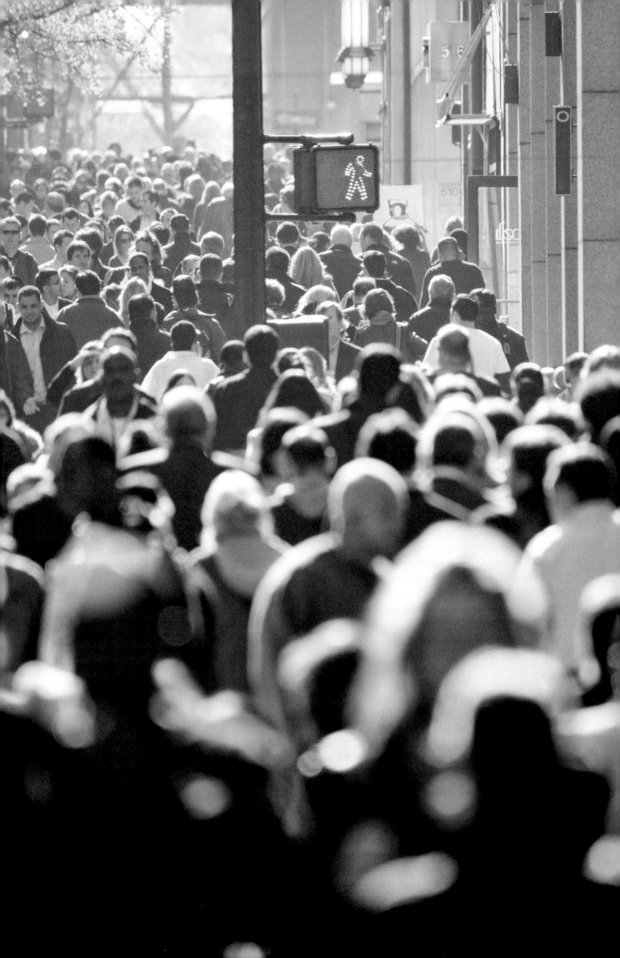

CHAPTER 2

A Disease of Epidemic Proportions

In the last ten years or so, it has become obvious that the number of patients with Alzheimer's disease is increasing. To fully understand the situation, we need to take a look at human life expectancy over the last two thousand years.

Figure 4 shows a curve depicting changes in the life expectancy of human beings since the beginning of the Christian era, nearly two thousand years ago. As we can see, in the time of Pontius Pilate and Jesus the average life expectancy barely reached the thirties (Wilmoth, 2000) — which paradoxically makes Jesus a rather active senior citizen of the time. It would take more than eighteen hundred years before there would be a slight increase in life expectancy in Europe. On the other hand, between 1800 and 2000, life expectancy increased significantly, almost doubling in less than two hundred years (Wilmoth, 2000, Fig. 4).

LIFE EXPECTANCY OVER THE CENTURIES

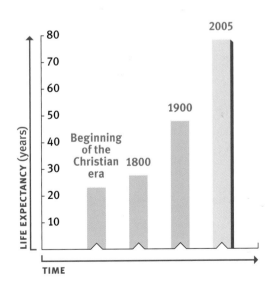

FIGURE 4

www.aaa.org, Statistics Canada, Dr. Judes Poirier

This explosion in the number of elderly people can be attributed mainly to the discovery of antibiotics and vaccines, a general improvement in hygiene, and a better diet, especially in the last century.

Since age (or aging, to be precise) is now considered to be the main risk factor for Alzheimer's disease (Gauthier, 2007), it goes without saying that a direct consequence of an increase in life expectancy was the revelation of how prevalent this terrible disease is, particularly in our western societies. At the same time, scientists have noted that the proportion of women likely to develop the disease increased significantly during the second half of the twentieth century. Today, roughly two-thirds of patients with Alzheimer's disease are women. We will examine a little later the underlying explanations for this somewhat surprising situation.

Figure 5 illustrates the breakdown by gender among people with the most common chronic diseases in western countries. The figure shows that more men than women (approximately two-thirds of patients) suffer from heart disease, cancer, and diabetes, while more women (approximately two-thirds of patients) are affected by dementias like Alzheimer's.

According to the most recent data from the World Health Organization (WHO), a new case of Alzheimer's occurs every seven seconds worldwide. In North America, it is estimated that there are more than 5.8 million patients with Alzheimer's disease (Alzheimer Disease International, 2010). In Europe, the number of old people with Alzheimer's disease exceeds six million cases, with Germany, Italy, and France at the top of

THE MOST COMMON CHRONIC DISEASES BY GENDER

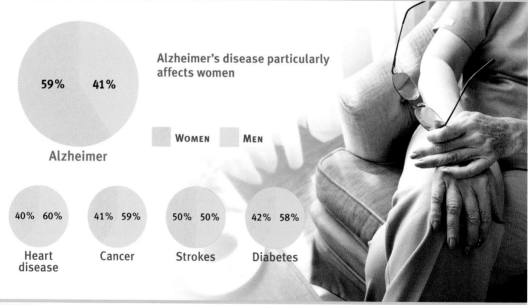

FIGURE 5

the list, the latter currently having more than 900,000 cases. Recent research findings from Asia indicate that there are more than six million cases in China alone. Figure 6 shows the most recent statistical analyses with respect to the West, and Figure 7 gives the most cautious projections, based on North American data, as to the number of cases expected by 2050.

Similar results were obtained in the twenty-five most populous European countries (www.alzheimer-europe.org). As can be seen, the predicted increase, based on the most recent data on baby boomers, raises the likelihood that the increase in the prevalence of Alzheimer's disease in the next forty years will reach near-epidemic proportions. In addition, it goes without saying that, in conjunction with this very dramatic worldwide upsurge in the disease, significant costs in the health sector are also to be expected in the coming years.

PREVALENCE OF ALZHEIMER'S DISEASE IN WESTERN COUNTRIES

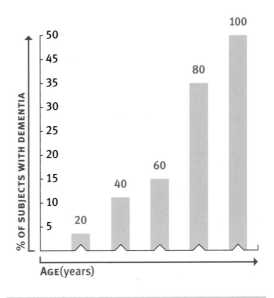

FIGURE 6   Source : Gauthier, 2006

PROJECTED PREVALENCE OF ALZHEIMER'S DISEASE IN NORTH AMERICA IN THE NEXT GENERATION

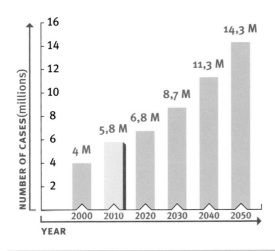

Currently 5.8 million cases

Over 14 million cases projected in a single generation

FIGURE 7   Source : www.alz.org

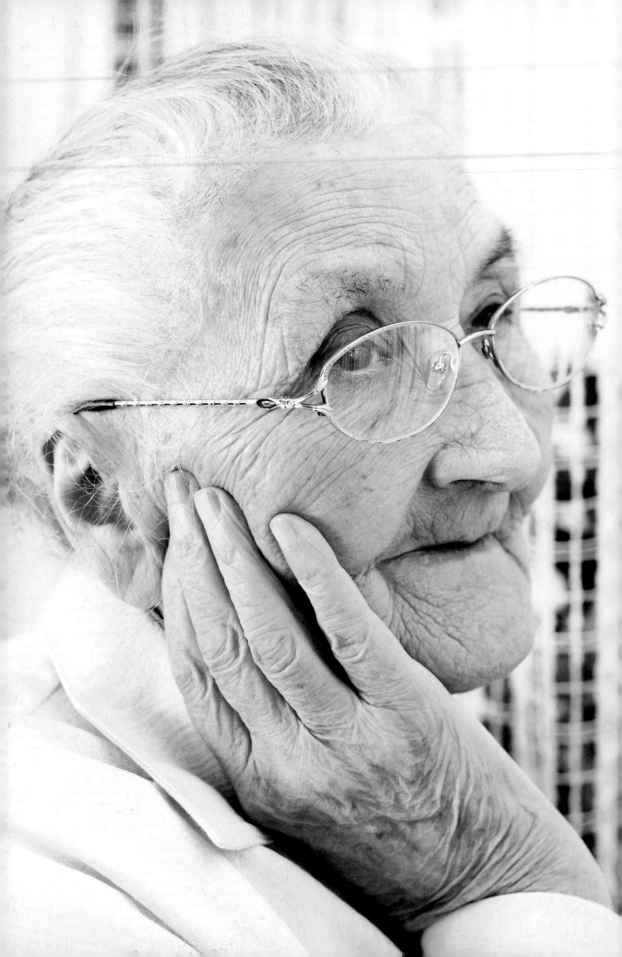

For instance, it has been determined that the annual direct and indirect costs associated with Alzheimer's disease in North America (Canada and the United States) now exceed 150 billion dollars (www.alz.org), which makes it one of the largest burdens on the health-care systems in these two countries. The forecasts for 2015, according to a recent study, are in the order of 195 billion dollars. In Europe, the direct costs associated with this disease are estimated at 52 billion euros per year; this does not include losses in productivity and the economic impact of the disease on informal caregivers (for indirect costs, go to www.alzheimer-europe.org). In light of this, given the enormous increase in the number of cases to come, it is easy to imagine the extent to which the disease will result in major expenditures and thus place a heavy load on our respective health-care systems.

A number of factors explain the explosion in the direct and indirect costs of Alzheimer's disease, especially in western countries. Drug prices, while high, represent only about 20 percent of the annual direct costs associated with Alzheimer's disease. Instead, it is the indirect expenses related to long-term care services that are a burden, because they are much higher for an Alzheimer's patient than for patients with other conditions. There is a very simple reason for this: it is estimated that a patient with Alzheimer's remains, on average, seven times longer in a long-term care facility than a patient suffering from neurological disorders not involving memory impairment.

Other indirect factors associated with Alzheimer's disease include work days missed, whether by an informal caregiver

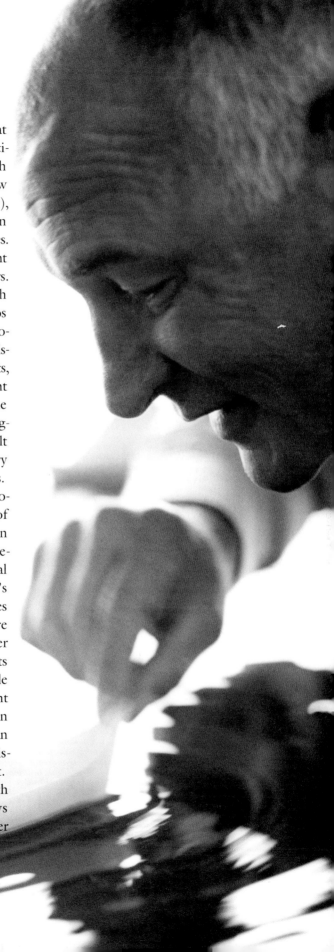

close to the patient or by the spouse, who must be available to help the patient and look after a large portion of his or her personal needs. It is important to understand that since roughly 70 percent of people with Alzheimer's disease live at home, the disease's impact goes far beyond the individual and often affects members of the immediate family, their friends, and even those responsible for providing day-to-day services.

For many years, the diseases most feared by the population in general were cancer, heart disease, stroke, and diabetes, respectively. However, the situation seems to have changed dramatically in the last decade, as indicated in a poll recently conducted in the United States, showing that Alzheimer's disease is now in second place among the diseases most feared by the general public (see Figure 9). What's more, when the respondents are over fifty-five, Alzheimer's disease replaces cancer; it

THE LARGE FAMILY OF DEMENTIAS AND ITS MAJOR SUB-GROUPS

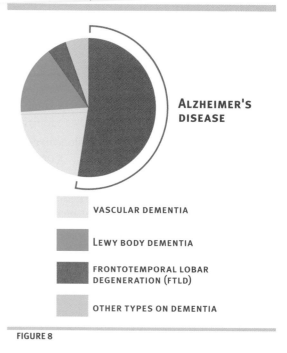

ALZHEIMER'S DISEASE

VASCULAR DEMENTIA

LEWY BODY DEMENTIA

FRONTOTEMPORAL LOBAR DEGENERATION (FTLD)

OTHER TYPES ON DEMENTIA

FIGURE 8

ANXIETY LEVELS IN THE NORTH AMERICAN POPULATION WITH RESPECT TO THE FIVE MAIN DISEASES

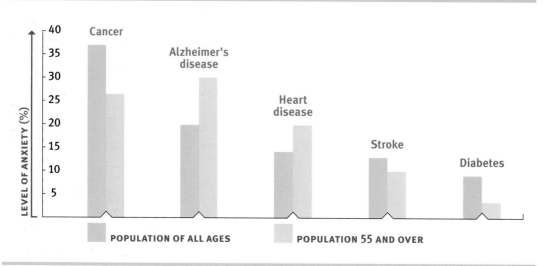

FIGURE 9

Source: www.alz.org

has been the major source of worry for this rapidly increasing group for many years now (www.alz.org).

In more general terms, Alzheimer's disease is part of the large family of dementias. The medical term "dementia" refers to a progressive loss of memory, as well as of certain intellectual abilities, to the point where this loss interferes with daily activities.

In the large family of dementias, Alzheimer's disease represents more than 60–70 percent of known and medically diagnosed cases. There are several other diseases also associated with memory loss,

confusion, and other symptoms usually attributed to dementia (see Figure 8).

These other diseases include "vascular" dementias (formerly called stroke-related dementias), characterized by a disruption in blood flow in the brain; "mixed" dementia, combining Alzheimer's disease and vascular dementia; "Parkinsonian" dementia, some of whose symptoms are similar to those of Parkinson's disease; and, lastly, "Lewy Body" dementia, which is strongly associated with attention deficits and hallucinations, as well as with a kind of muscular rigidity very similar to that seen in Parkinson's disease.

Alzheimer's Disease in Figures

Life expectancy has almost tripled in two thousand years and almost doubled in the last two hundred. Like other chronic diseases, dementia strikes twice as many women as men. The proportion of people with Alzheimer's disease increases from 6 to 8 percent among sixty-five-year-olds to more than 40 percent among people eighty and older. On the list of diseases causing concern in people fifty-five and older, Alzheimer's disease now comes first. The number of people with the disease will double in the space of one generation, affecting more than eighty million individuals worldwide, with a new case every seven seconds. In 2010, it was estimated that more than 600 billion dollars were being spent globally on patients with Alzheimer's disease.

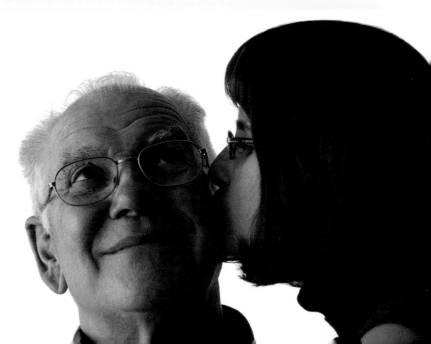

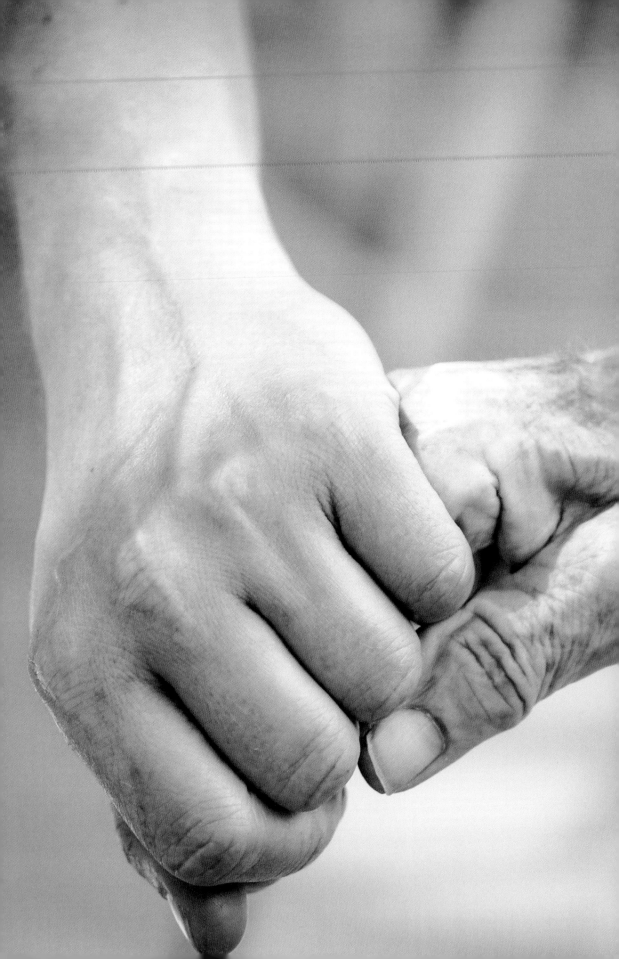

In Summary

A Disease of Epidemic Proportions

If we take into account the demographic changes now occurring in western societies, it is clear that, despite the staggering expenditures devoted collectively and individually to Alzheimer's disease, with the massive arrival of the baby boomer cohort in the vulnerable age range (60–70 years of age), we are currently seeing just the tip of an iceberg that the entire world will run aground on in less than a generation if nothing is done in the realm of scientific research. Fortunately, there have been significant advances in our understanding of the biology of the disease, as well as in therapeutic treatment. These advances have led to the discovery of effective symptomatic drugs, among other things, which do not, however, provide a cure for the disease. A shift in direction is needed; for several years, major investments in research have been called for, in both Europe and the United States, to give the engines of the large and small research centres working on dementia and its prevention a significant boost.

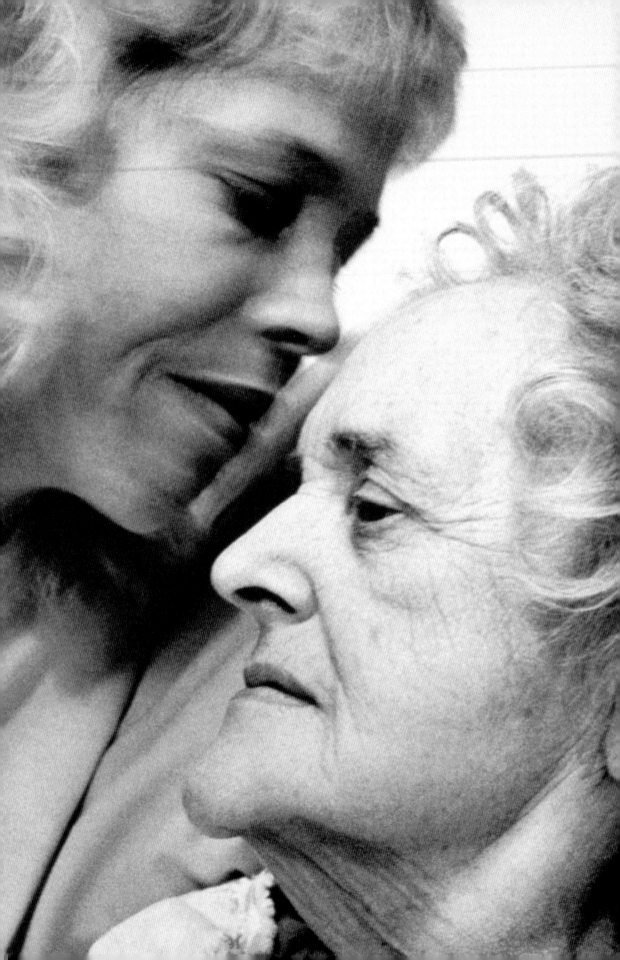

CHAPTER 3

Diagnosing Alzheimer's Disease

This chapter explains how a diagnosis of Alzheimer's disease is usually made. It also includes a description of new diagnostic tests being developed that could make early detection possible.

THE FIRST SYMPTOMS OF ALZHEIMER'S DISEASE

Most people with Alzheimer's disease complain about their memory for several months or years before their forgetfulness disturbs their professional and social lives in any significant way. For example, items get lost, meetings are missed, bills are paid late or twice, a stove burner is left on. Some people make light of these difficulties, while others worry a good deal about them. Most people with memory lapses do not have Alzheimer's disease, but occasional forgetfulness may indicate a risk for later on (see Chapter 7 on

prevention). For a diagnosis of Alzheimer's disease to be confirmed, there must be, in addition to memory loss, a decline in another area of intellectual activity, usually language and (or) judgement and decision-making. The combination of a recent decline in memory and changes in another intellectual sphere, coupled with a decreasing ability to carry out day-to-day activities, indicates a dementia whose cause has to be determined: Alzheimer's disease, stroke, Parkinson's disease, or a combination of the three.

The doctor being consulted must, with the help of family, a friend, or a neighbour, ask the person questions about his or her usual daily activities. These questions differ for men and women, working or retired people, and younger or older people. Figure 10 gives a list of daily activities affected by Alzheimer's disease as it progresses. This list is based on the *Disability Assessment for Dementia*, or DAD, developed by Louise

DAY-TO-DAY ACTIVITIES AFFECTED BY ALZHEIMER'S DISEASE

- Preparing meals
- Making phone calls
- Going out
- Managing finances and correspondence
- Taking medication properly
- Participating in leisure activities and carrying out domestic tasks
- Personal grooming
- Getting dressed
- Eating
- Exercising bladder and bowel control

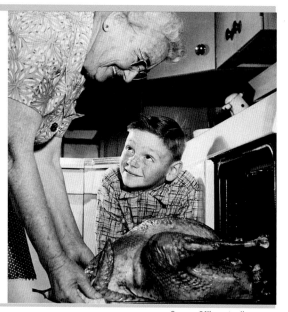

FIGURE 10

Source : Gélinas et coll., 1999

BEHAVIOURAL DISORDERS IN ALZHEIMER'S DISEASE IN ORDER OF FREQUENCY

Gauthier's team in Montreal. Research conducted in France by a team under Dr. François Dartigues has shown that the four activities most frequently impaired right at the outset of Alzheimer's disease are the safe use of drugs, efficient use of transportation, regular use of the telephone or another means of communication, and responsible management of finances. Social withdrawal is often a result of difficulties in using transportation and communicating, combined with apathy, which is the first and most frequent of the behavioural symptoms associated with Alzheimer's disease. Figure 11 lists behaviours seen in the various stages of Alzheimer's disease, in order of frequency. This list is based on the *Neuropsychiatric Inventory,* or NPI, developed by Dr. Jeffrey Cummings in Los Angeles.

- Apathy
- Agitation
- Motor activity
- Aberrant behaviours (night-time)
- Depression
- Appetite changes
- Anxiety
- Irritability
- Delusions
- Lack of inhibition
- Hallucinations
- Euphoria

FIGURE 11

Source : Cummings et al., 1997

CRITERIA FOR ESTABLISHING A DIAGNOSIS OF "PROBABLE" ALZHEIMER'S DISEASE

- Cognitive decline
- Functional impairment
- Absence of any other brain or systemic disease to explain symptoms

FIGURE 12   Source : McKhann et al., revised 2011

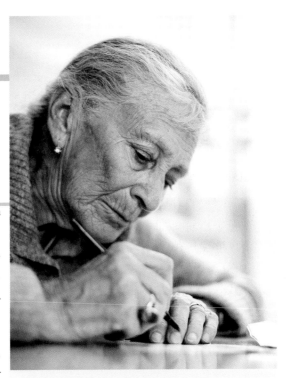

Variations in the clinical presentation of Alzheimer's disease are possible: frequently searching for words (aphasia), having misconceptions about people or thinking you are being watched (paranoia), and displaying uninhibited social behaviour. These variations affect our degree of certainty about the cause of the symptoms. The diagnosis of Alzheimer's disease has an accuracy rate of 85–90 percent when the presentation is classic ("probable" Alzheimer's disease, a diagnosis based on criteria developed by McKhann et al., and summarized in Figure 12).

It is important to check the entire medical history to see if there are any factors contributing to memory decline, in particular depression, overuse of tranquillizers, sleep apnea, deafness, and vision loss.

WHAT ARE THE TESTS FOR A PERSON SUSPECTED OF HAVING ALZHEIMER'S DISEASE?

The physician or a member of the medical team will administer simple cognitive tests such as the *Mini Mental State Examination* (MMSE) developed in New York

A Typical Case History of the Onset of Alzheimer's Disease

Mrs. Wilson is eighty-four years old. She has lived alone since her husband's death ten years ago. Her daughter has noticed that her mother calls less often and has stopped going to choir practice, although she used to really enjoy it. Unpaid bills are piling up in a drawer. The fridge contains stale food. When her daughter visited and shared her concerns, Mrs. Wilson got angry. She blamed the neighbour, claiming she had stolen a piece of jewellery she couldn't find.

A brain scan without contrast (computed tomography or CT scan, or computerized axial tomography (CAT scan) is most often done to make sure there is no tumour, no excess fluid in the ventricles or subdural hematoma (very rare), and that no small strokes have occurred (fairly common).

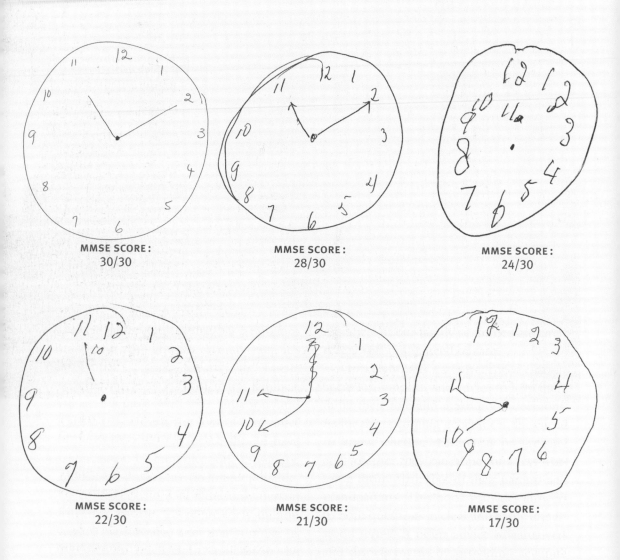

MMSE SCORE:
30/30

MMSE SCORE:
28/30

MMSE SCORE:
24/30

MMSE SCORE:
22/30

MMSE SCORE:
21/30

MMSE SCORE:
17/30

Examples of clocks drawn respectively by a person without Alzheimer's disease and people at various stages of cognitive impairment, based on MMSE test scores

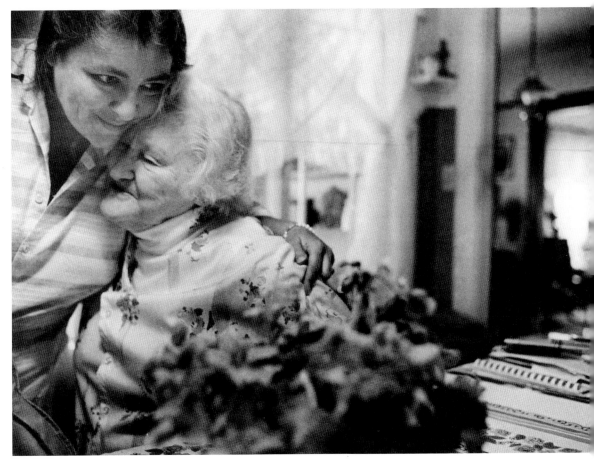

by Dr. Barry Reisberg, which does not provide a diagnosis per se, but measures certain aspects of the person's intellectual functioning: orientation in time and space, the ability to remember three words, and to spell, read, write, and copy a drawing. The result, out of a total of thirty points, may be influenced by the level of education and nervousness.

When the test is normal (greater than twenty-six out of thirty), it is now routine to administer the *Montreal Cognitive Assessment* (MoCA), designed by Dr. Ziad Nasreddine, which takes a more in-depth look at what are called "executive" intellectual abilities and includes having the person draw a clock and testing his or her delayed recall of five words (also rated out of thirty). Examples of clocks supposed to show 11:10 are on page 42.

If these tests are normal, but memory complaints have the potential to significantly disrupt the person's work, an in-depth neuropsychological evaluation done by a psychologist may be requested to examine memory, language, and the skills used to make decisions or adapt to new situations.

A general health assessment is then carried out, including a blood test to see if the person is anaemic, has a thyroid, liver, or kidney problems, or a vitamin deficiency, especially B12. There is at present no routine genetic test for diagnosing Alzheimer's disease.

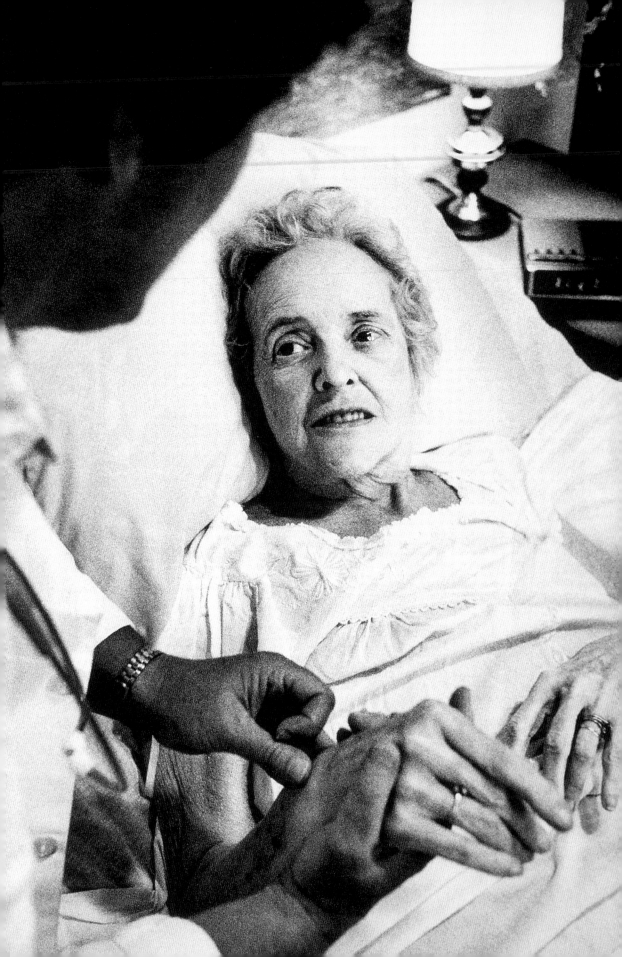

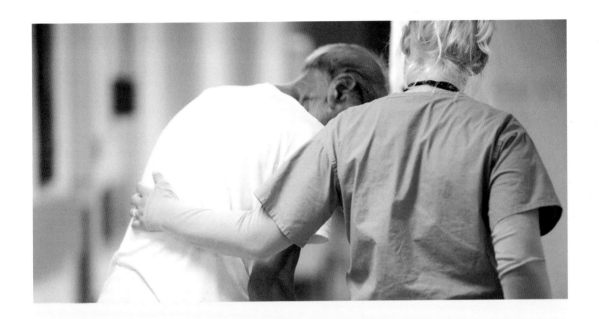

An Example of Assessment by a Family Doctor

Mrs. Wilson has agreed to go to the doctor so her daughter will "leave her alone." After a review of the symptoms, the family history is examined: her mother was confused in the final years of her life and died at ninety-two. There is no obvious depression. She does not take any drugs, other than calcium supplements. Her MMSE score of nineteen out of thirty is abnormal for someone with seven years of education. She gets the day, date, month, year, city, country, place name, and floor wrong, she forgets two out of three words and cannot copy the drawing of two overlapping pentagons. In addition, she is unable to draw a clock showing 11:10. Her blood profile is normal, except for the level of Vitamin B12, which is slightly below normal. Her brain scan shows normal atrophy for her age and a few ischemic changes around the ventricles (see Figure 14).

The MMSE test is re-administered two months later and the result is now eighteen out of thirty.

An example of the appropriate way to tell the patient her test results

Mrs. Wilson wants to know what is happening to her.

"Is it the same disease my mother had?" she asks.

"Perhaps," says the doctor. "Your memory lapses are due to aging of the brain, as there are no signs of blood clots on the scan. Aside from a slightly low level of Vitamin B12, your general health is good. Would you agree to having an occupational therapist from the CLSC visit you at home to make sure everything is safe?"

A differential diagnosis for Alzheimer's disease takes into account all of the symptoms and abnormalities found during the examination. Alzheimer's disease is often associated with atherosclerosis of the brain or with a low level of Vitamin B12 in the blood. This does not alter the main diagnosis, namely, Alzheimer's disease. There may also be slight depression, especially in the early stage of the disease.

WHAT THE DOCTOR TELLS A DIAGNOSED PATIENT

A trusted person (a spouse or child) is usually informed as soon as possible that Alzheimer's disease is a possibility. The patient will be told that there is a serious medical problem and will be congratulated for having come for advice early on, ensuring that the memory problem can be treated immediately, perhaps preventing complications. The words "dementia" and "Alzheimer's" are avoided, unless the patient asks a very specific question. In that case, an honest response is given, unless there is the likelihood of a catastrophic reaction. A trusting doctor–patient relationship is preferable to a secretive one, as decisions must be made quite quickly to choose a proxy in case of incapacity, in the presence of a notary or a lawyer; the proxy will also be given a general power of attorney.

Financial security, whether the person can or cannot drive a car or get around alone on public transport, and the use of kitchen equipment must all be assessed. A safety assessment scale has been developed by Dr. Louise Poulin de Courval and her team in Montreal (see Figure 13) to help make the assessment, which can assist in determining whether the person needs supervision at home.

SAFETY ASSESSMENT SCALE

- Informal caregiver and environment
- Use of tobacco
- Fire and burns
- Nutrition
- Food poisoning and toxic substances
- Medication and health problems
- Wandering and adaptation to temperature changes

FIGURE 13   Source : Poulin de Courval et al., 2006

EXAMPLE OF BRAIN IMAGING

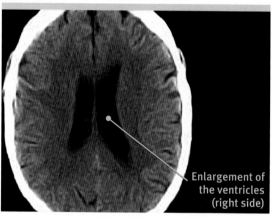

Enlargement of the ventricles (right side)

Computed tomography (CT scan) typical of a person with Alzheimer's disease (early stage) with mild global atrophy and a few ischemic changes around the lateral ventricles.

FIGURE 14

DOES A SPECIALIST HAVE TO BE CONSULTED?

Family doctors have been trained to diagnose Alzheimer's disease and manage its treatment. Checking the diagnosis by consulting a spe-

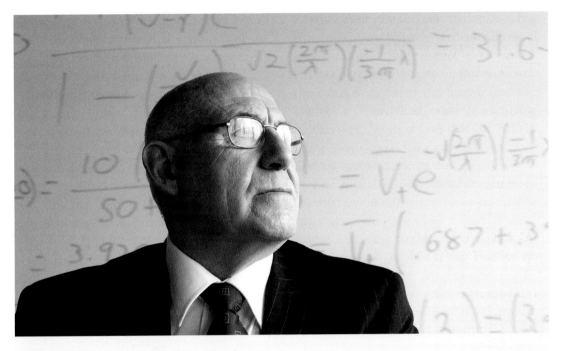

The Story of an Individual who consults a Specialist about his Memory

Dr. Taylor is a university professor. He is sixty-four and worried about his memory — he is having trouble preparing his courses and remembering the names of his students. Sometimes he loses the thread of his ideas in class and he is depending more and more on his notes. His mother died of Alzheimer's disease at sixty-six. He gets twenty-nine out of thirty on his MMSE test, and twenty-six out of thirty on his MoCA test. He is therefore referred for neuropsychological tests, which reveal a significant short-term memory deficit in comparison with his age group and education level. The MRI indicates atrophy in the hippocampus and the FDG-PET shows a metabolic decline in the parietal and cingulate regions. The specialist diagnoses early-stage Alzheimer's disease.

Dr. Taylor wants to know his diagnosis so he can stop working early and enjoy his retirement. The university and the government pension board accept his disability claim.

cialist — a neurologist, geriatric psychiatrist, or geriatrician — is recommended, if the person affected is young at the onset of the disease (under sixty-five), there is uncertainty about the diagnosis, there is no significant response to the usual treatment, or the patient wants to participate in research.

The specialist will take the medical history again, redo the physical examination, and make sure that blood tests and a brain scan have been done. In some cases, additional brain scans will be requested: 1) a magnetic resonance imaging test (MRI) to detect any generalized or focal atrophy,

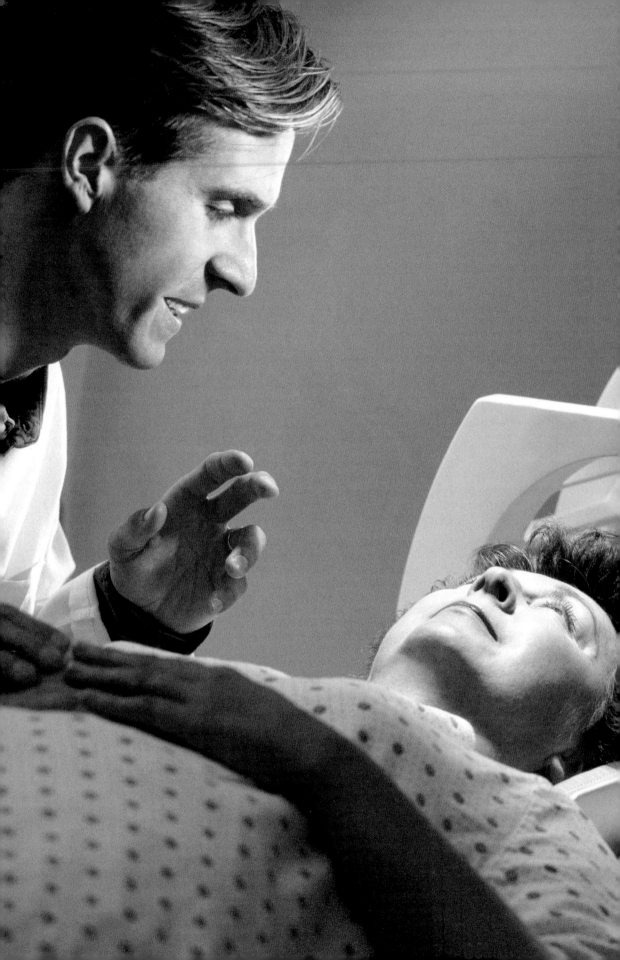

and any small infarcts in some regions known to be "strategic" for memory, such as the thalamus or the head of the caudate nucleus, and 2) fluorodeoxyglucose–positron emission tomography (FDG-PET), to see if this radioactive sugar is being metabolized consistently in the various regions of the brain.

An MRI in the presence of Alzheimer's disease shows atrophy of the entire brain (Figure 15, left) but especially in the hippocampus region (Figure 15, right). The FDG-PET will show a decline in metabolism (thus indirectly a decrease in the number of nerve cells and their connections and synapses) in the posterior regions of the brain (Figure 16, top and centre) and in the posterior cingulum (Figure 16, bottom).

A combination of memory tests, an MRI, and a PET could make it possible to diagnose Alzheimer's disease while the symptoms are still very mild. In some countries, a lumbar puncture (LP) is also done to measure the level in the cerebrospinal fluid of two proteins whose levels are abnormal right from the onset of Alzheimer's disease: beta-amyloid, which is low, and tau, which is generally high. A PET using a marker for amyloid, the protein that accumulates in the brain of everyone with Alzheimer's disease, is currently under development (PIB scan). All of the brain scans now available to establish a diagnosis of Alzheimer's disease are summarized in Figure 17. A group of researchers under the direction of Dr. Bruno Dubois, in Paris, have suggested that these

EXAMPLES OF ATROPHIED BRAINS

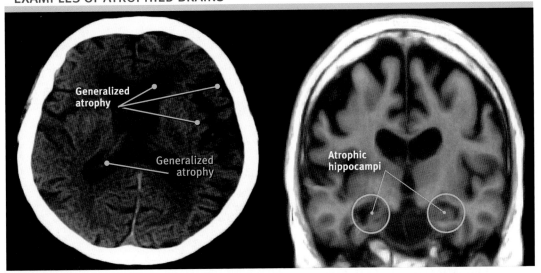

Magnetic resonance imaging (MRI) of a brain with Alzheimer's disease
Horizontal view showing a brain with global atrophy

Magnetic resonance imaging (MRI) of a brain with Alzheimer's disease
Coronal view showing atrophic hippocampi

FIGURE 15

FLUORODEOXYGLUCOSE-POSITRON EMISSION TOMOGRAPHY (FDG-PET) OF A BRAIN WITH ALZHEIMER'S DISEASE

Magnetic resonance
(control subject)

Healthy brain
(control subject)

Brain with
Alzheimer's Disease

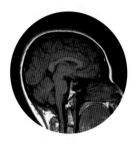
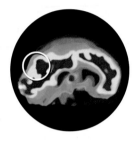
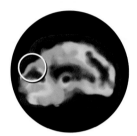

SAGITTAL
VIEW

Hypometabolism in
the posterior cingulum

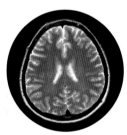
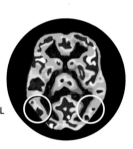

HORIZONTAL
VIEW

Hypometabolism in
the parietotemporal regions

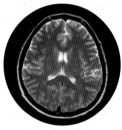
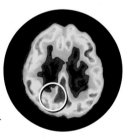
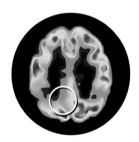

HORIZONTAL
VIEW

Hypometabolism in
the parietotemporal regions

Metabolism [^{18}F]FDG

Minimum -   + Maximum

FIGURE 16

tests (brain scans and the examination of the cerebrospinal fluid) are in themselves sufficient to make an early diagnosis of Alzheimer's disease, even if memory lapses are the only problem — a stage known as "predementia" Alzheimer's disease.

This kind of situation is quite rare, as the majority of patients with Alzheimer's disease are already retired. That said, diagnosis is urgently required for health professionals (doctors, nurses, pharmacists), people who manage finances, or anyone for whom forgetting things or making errors in judgement in their work may have unfortunate consequences for others and for themselves. On the other hand, a very early diag-

nosis is not without risk — as the person will understand everything the diagnosis implies, this may cause a catastrophic reaction. For the time being, there is no available treatment at this stage of Alzheimer's disease and supplementary tests (MRI and FDG-PET) are expensive. Researchers such as Dr. Serge Gauthier in Montreal and Dr. Philip Scheltens in Amsterdam have recommended that information on the results of diagnostic tests be given gradually to patients, after the risk of a catastrophic reaction has been assessed, and that this type of very early diagnosis not be made widely available as long as the possibility of participating in therapeutic research does not exist.

CEREBRAL SCANS USED IN THE DIAGNOSIS OF ALZHEIMER'S DISEASE

Computerized axial tomography (CAT or CT scan)	Basic examination to eliminate the possibility of strokes, tumours, hematomas, and hydrocephalus.
Magnetic resonance imaging (MRI)	More specialized examination to detect the presence of ischemic changes smaller than a stroke and atrophy in the regions of the brain related to memory (hippocampi, temporal lobes). If it is repeated, the rate of atrophy of the entire brain can be measured (normally 1 percent per year!).
Fluorodeoxyglucose-positron emission tomography (FDG-PET)	Specialized examination to assess the metabolism of brain regions by comparing them with each other. In Alzheimer's disease, there is early hypometabolism (sometimes before symptoms appear) in the parietotemporal regions and the posterior cingulum.
Positron emission tomography with injection of a product that chemically binds with amyloid fibrils, for example, the Pittsburgh Compound (PIB-PET)	In the case of Alzheimer's disease, this test reveals a higher level of deposits in the anterior regions of the brain several years before symptoms appear.

FIGURE 17

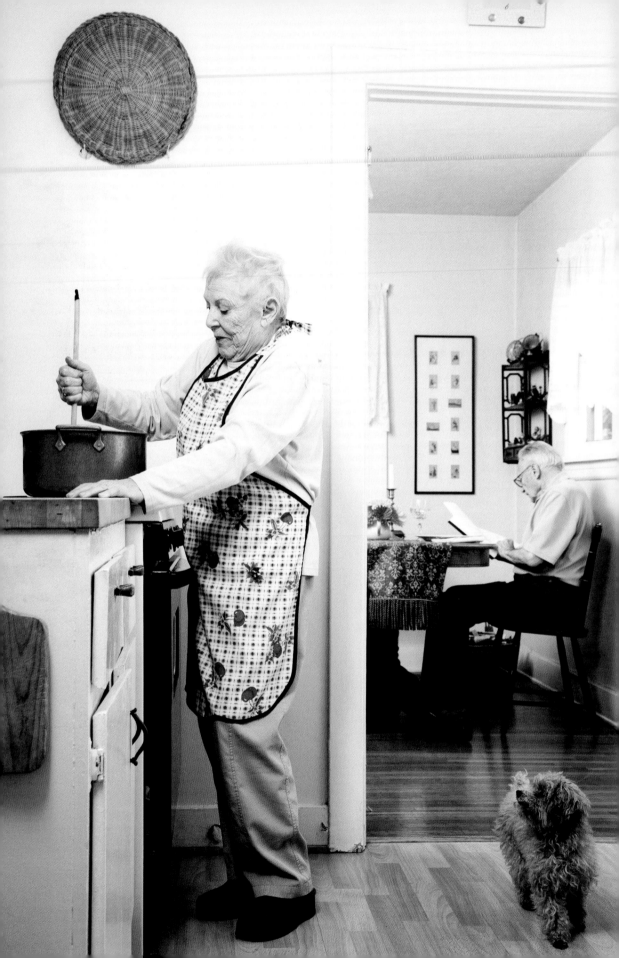

In Summary

Diagnosing Alzheimer's Disease

A diagnosis of Alzheimer's disease is made by a family doctor, sometimes in conjunction with a specialist. The diagnosis is 85 percent accurate when the symptoms are typical: a gradual decline in short-term memory, other intellectual impairment, and difficulty in carrying out daily activities. The evaluation is simple in most cases, consisting of an MMSE test, blood tests, and computerized axial tomography (CAT scan). When the symptoms are very mild but it is urgent to make a diagnosis, additional tests — neuropsychology, MRI, FDG-PET, and lumbar puncture — are required.

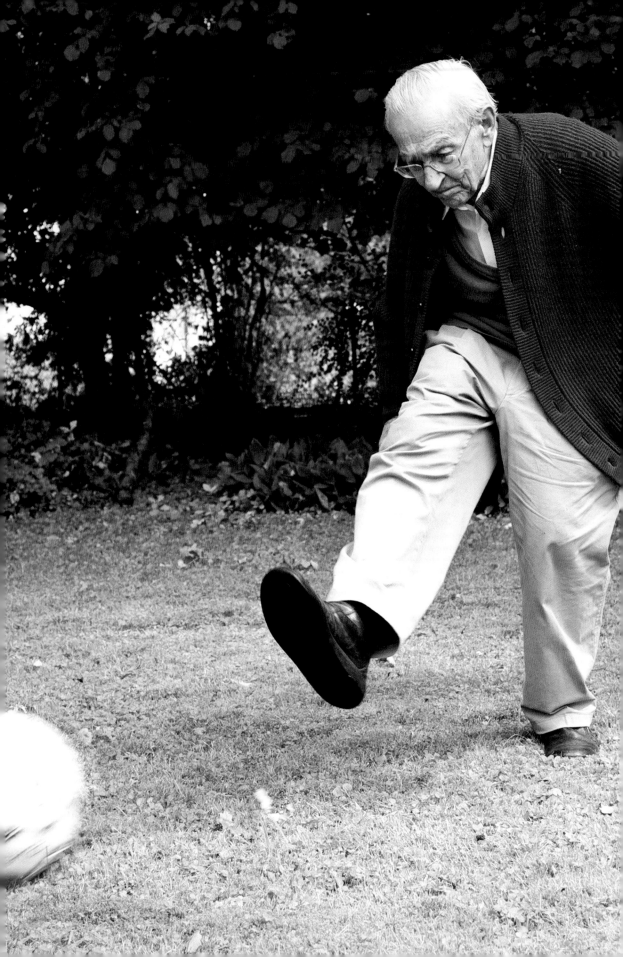

CHAPTER 4

The Natural Progression of Alzheimer's Disease

Traditionally, Alzheimer's disease was diagnosed when there were enough symptoms to indicate "dementia" and the most probable cause was more likely to be Alzheimer's disease than a stroke or Parkinson's disease. However, the symptoms that precede dementia are often subtle and develop slowly. This is why researchers are more and more interested in the stage of Alzheimer's disease called "predemential" or "prodromal," in which early treatment to stop or slow down the progression of the disease might be possible. Once dementia has taken hold, its progression is more or less predictable over eight to ten years — hence the importance of being familiar with the natural progression of Alzheimer's disease so as to anticipate the stages that lie ahead. This chapter describes the progression of the disease from beginning to end, providing a better understanding of the current and developing treatments discussed in later chapters.

THE STAGES OF ALZHEIMER'S DISEASE

The classification system most often used worldwide is the *Global Deterioration Scale* (GDS) developed by Dr. Barry Reisberg in New York, consisting of seven stages (Figure 18).

Stage 1 applies to everyone who ages normally, but also to people who are likely to develop Alzheimer's disease at some point. The degree of risk varies greatly from one individual to another depending on family history (genetic baggage) and what happens to that person in the course of a lifetime (level of education, high blood pressure, etc.). A later chapter will describe how we can determine the risk of getting Alzheimer's disease later in life and how a "primary" preventive approach is being developed.

Stage 2 of the disease is characterized by "subjective cognitive impairment" or

SCI. The impression that our brain is slowing down is very familiar to all of us, especially after fifty. After this age, learning a new language becomes difficult (although not impossible), we adapt to change more slowly, and we forget the names of people we know. All of this is normal. However, if people who have been engaged in activities of a certain intellectual calibre notice a slowing down at work or in their complex leisure activities (playing bridge, for example) in a relatively short period (approximately a year), this should be looked into by their family doctor. Most people with symptoms of this kind do not end up with Alzheimer's disease; however, this could be an opportunity for "secondary" prevention of the disease, since the individual already has symptoms.

Stage 3 has been the object of the most research for the last five to seven years since, in this stage, very early treatment to interrupt or slow down the progression of Alzheimer's disease may be possible. It is usually referred to as "mild cognitive impairment" or MCI. In this stage, depending on the person's age, genetic baggage, and other biological markers under development (see Chapter 3 on diagnosis), the progression towards Alzheimer's disease is in the order of 15 percent per year for five years (or 75 percent risk), after which the risk decreases (Figure 19). Some epidemiological studies carried out in large populations suggest that the majority (over 90 percent) of people in stage 3 do not deteriorate further and may even return to normal. There is therefore a need to specify and validate the criteria for diagnosing very early stage Alzheimer's disease, as proposed by Mayeux and his colleagues in 2011. However, many experimental treatments are tested in stage 3 on people who have been diagnosed with very early stage Alzheimer's disease — in other words, who have no significant functional problems or dementia.

Stage 4 is where Alzheimer's disease is usually recognized by everyone (family, friends, neighbours), but often denied by the person affected. This "anosognosia,"

REISBERG'S GLOBAL DETERIORATION SCALE

Stage 1	No symptoms
Stage 2	Mild symptoms (short-term memory lapses, difficulty making decisions) with no measurable decline on neuropsychological tests
Stage 3	Mild symptoms with measurable decline on neuropsychological tests, but with no significant effect on day-to-day activities
Stage 4	Mild dementia (ability to drive a car as long as accompanied by someone)
Stage 5	Moderate dementia (choice of clothing made by someone else; gets around on foot in familiar places only; finances managed by another person)
Stage 6	Severe dementia (must be washed and dressed by another person; cannot be left alone)
Stage 7	Very severe to end-stage dementia (inability to walk safely; difficulty swallowing)

FIGURE 18

Source: Reisberg et coll., 1984

or the lack of awareness by the individual of his or her functional difficulties, makes the burden slightly lighter for the person, but not for the family. The person can usually drive a car in familiar locations and carry out simple and routine tasks and cook for him or herself, but not for an entire visiting family. The person needs advice on complicated financial decisions, but can go alone to the wicket at the bank (not to the automatic banking machine) to make a deposit or withdrawal.

Stage 5, or "moderate dementia," is where the need for personal care becomes obvious: someone has to choose the patient's clothes or suggest taking a shower. Driving a car becomes impossible and out-ings on foot are limited to the immediate vicinity, unless the person wears an identifi-cation bracelet. Behavioural symptoms like irritability may appear. Often, the caregiver gets in touch with the Alzheimer's Society to attend information sessions or join a support group. It becomes difficult to leave the sick person alone at home, as he or she might leave a burner on the stove turned on, a tap running, or a door open or unlocked.

In stage 6, or "severe dementia," it becomes increasingly difficult to function and behavioural problems such as "aggres-siveness and agitation" appear, especially when it is time to bathe or in the evening (Sundowners Syndrome). The person may no longer recognize a spouse, which sometimes causes crises where the latter is pushed out of bed, the bedroom, or even the house. Responsibilities increase for family members who, at this stage, will seek outside help for bathing and home care and think seriously about long-term residential care.

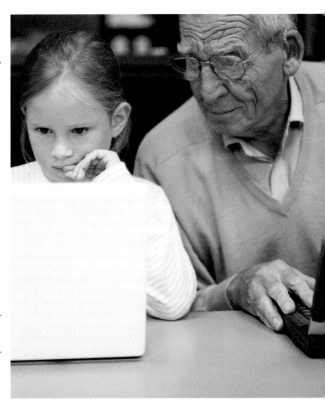

PREVALENCE OF STAGE 3 (OR MILD COGNITIVE IMPAIRMENT) AT VARIOUS AGES AFTER 70

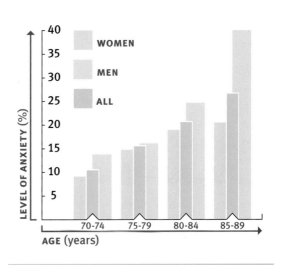

FIGURE 19   Source : www.alz.org

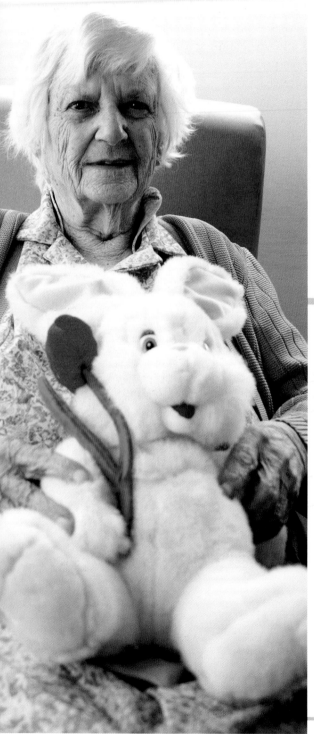

Stage 7, known as "very severe to late-stage," is characterized by total dependence in all aspects of daily life. Changes in motor abilities affect balance in walking, with the person gradually confined to a wheelchair, a geriatric chair, and then a bed. Verbal language disappears, although non-verbal communication (reaction to touch or tone of voice) remains present for a long time. The patient has trouble swallowing (dysphagia) and chokes while drinking and eating, which leads to aspiration pneumonia, the usual cause of death, occurring eight to ten years after stage 3 (Figure 20).

BRAIN CELL LOSS IN VARIOUS REGIONS OF THE BRAIN

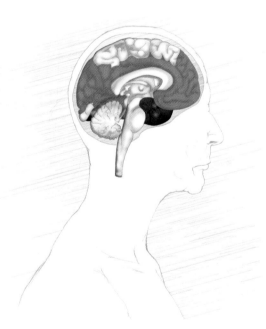

By stages 6 and 7, the disease has invaded almost the entire brain, especially the regions for memory and learning (in red).

FIGURE 20

THE IMMEDIATE IMPACT OF ALZHEIMER'S DISEASE AS IT PROGRESSES

DRIVING A CAR

Usually, driving in stage 4 of Alzheimer's disease poses few problems, as long as the person stays on well-known routes. Bringing someone along to act as "navigator" is recommended by the doctor and sometimes required by the motor vehicle licensing body.

In stage 5, a person is rarely authorized to drive a car, unless he or she can pass a road test with an occupational therapist or another qualified examiner and is always accompanied by another adult.

Losing a driver's licence is often a painful experience for a person who is ill and, by extension, for the whole family. Some patients will not forgive the doctor for submitting a report to the motor vehicle licence issuing body. Sometimes, the person is referred to a specialist specifically so he or she can be declared unfit to drive, thus protecting the therapeutic relationship between the person and the family doctor. Everyone with Alzheimer's disease will one day have to stop driving; it is possible to prepare for this stage of the disease with the family, sometimes by encouraging the partner to learn to drive, moving closer to public transportation, or creating a larger social network in which to find volunteer drivers.

WORKING OUTSIDE THE HOME

In stage 3, everyone is self-sufficient and independent in their usual daily activities. However, professionals (for example, doctors, nurses, pharmacists, lawyers, accountants, and teachers) with significant social responsibilities may have to stop working because of the risk of making professional errors. A neurological evaluation during which special attention is paid to working memory and executive abilities is usually required and sometimes repeated six to twelve months later. New diagnostic criteria for very early stage Alzheimer's disease suggested by Dubois and his colleagues (2007, 2010) and outlined in the preceding chapter, in addition to the use of brain imaging, could make it easier to obtain a disability report for medical reasons. In contrast, people who do manual or routine work with no danger to themselves

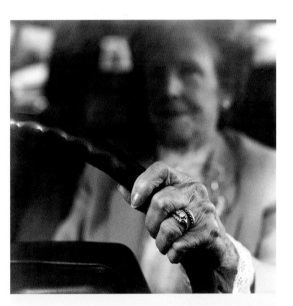

Driving with Alzheimer's Disease

Mrs. Johnson is in the habit of using her car to go and visit her daughter. To do this, she has to take the highway and cross a bridge. One day, because of roadwork, the bridge is closed and she has to make a detour. Mrs. Johnson gets lost and has to phone home to get directions.

ABILITY TO ACTIVATE THE BRAIN

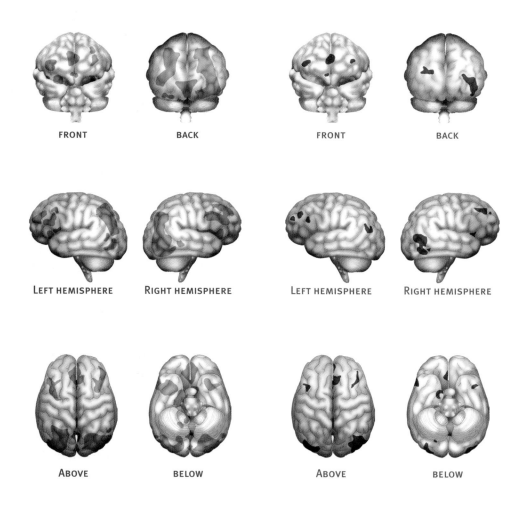

FRONT   BACK   FRONT   BACK

LEFT HEMISPHERE   RIGHT HEMISPHERE   LEFT HEMISPHERE   RIGHT HEMISPHERE

ABOVE   BELOW   ABOVE   BELOW

Normal brains

Brains with stage 3
Alzheimer's disease

During an exercise involving recognizing familiar objects, a significant decrease in the ability to activate the brain regions responsible for memory and learning is observed.

FIGURE 21   Source : le Dr Davis Knopman, Mayo Clinic, Rochester (New York)

or others can continue in stages 3 and 4 without changing tasks. Furthermore, the social interaction that is part of working is therapeutic for people. Even in stage 5, some patients continue to visit the site of the family business to maintain contact with the oldest clients and stay in touch with their former life.

EXECUTING LEGAL DOCUMENTS

The drafting of a general power of attorney and a health-care proxy in case of incapacity, with the help of a lawyer or notary, is strongly recommended before stage 5. The designated substitute decision-maker will thus be able to offer a person with Alzheimer's disease increasing assistance in managing his or her finances and making decisions about medical care. It is possible (and desirable) to appoint two substitute decision-makers to share the task. Otherwise, a replacement substitute decision-maker must be named in case the first is not able to fulfil this role.

Writing or changing a will is more complicated than choosing a substitute decision-maker. And whatever the stage of Alzheimer's disease, there is a risk it will be contested by a family member unhappy with the way the inheritance is divided after the person's death. To avoid this situation, it is wise to have a special assessment done by an expert to determine the person's competence to make a will, thus reducing the risk of costly litigation later on.

When a health-care proxy in case of incapacity is being drawn up, it is a good idea to specify the person's preferences for various options in situations that will arise in the course of Alzheimer's disease: participation in medical research (spec-ify if the person is interested and, if so, what degree of risk is acceptable), feeding if swallowing becomes difficult, and how to treat pneumonia if there is no longer any quality of life. The substitute decision-maker will have the last word when these decisions have to be made, but the task will be easier if the Alzheimer's patient has indicated his or her preferences beforehand.

Alzheimer's and Finances

Mr. White can no longer reliably write and sign cheques and a stranger borrowed five hundred dollars from him in cash. Mr. White's daughter asks the family doctor what can be done to protect her father's assets.

Work and Social Life after the Onset of Alzheimer's Disease

Mrs. Macdonald has always worked in the family grocery store. She can no longer calculate the clients' change, but she likes to spend the day chatting with clients she has known for a long time.

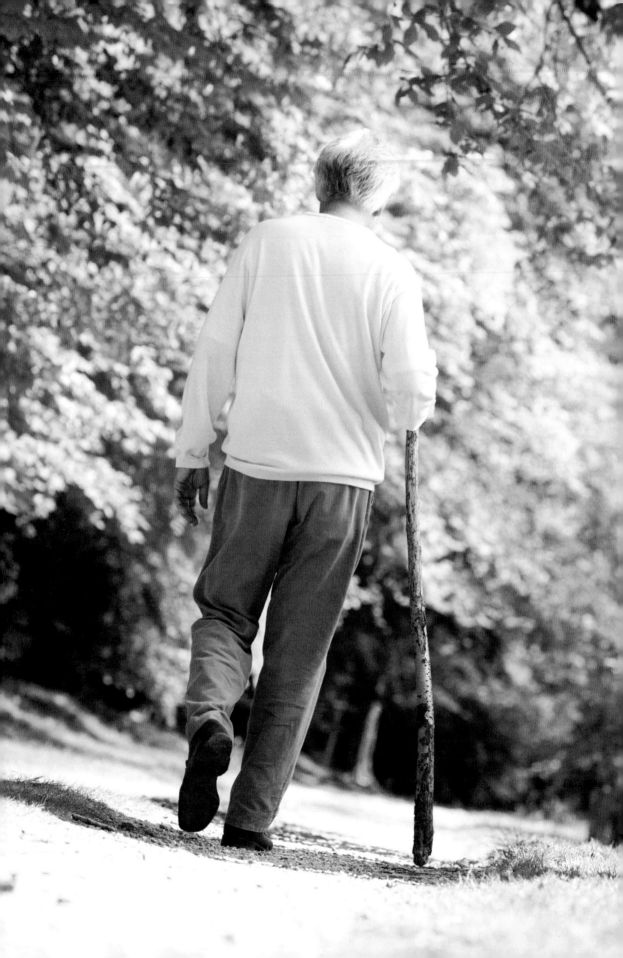

In Summary

The Natural Progression of Alzheimer's Disease

The seven stages of Alzheimer's disease are useful benchmarks both for research and in clinical practice with patients. They make it possible to assess the affected person's ability to carry out everyday activities. The ability to drive a car must be assessed periodically. Whether the person can continue to work regularly depends on his or her responsibilities and the consequences of potential errors at work. Drawing up a health-care proxy in case of incapacity and a general power of attorney is recommended as soon as Alzheimer's disease is diagnosed. It is desirable to indicate the person's preferences with regard to treating the disease, especially in its advanced stages. Lastly, if changes must be made to a will, a specialized assessment is required.

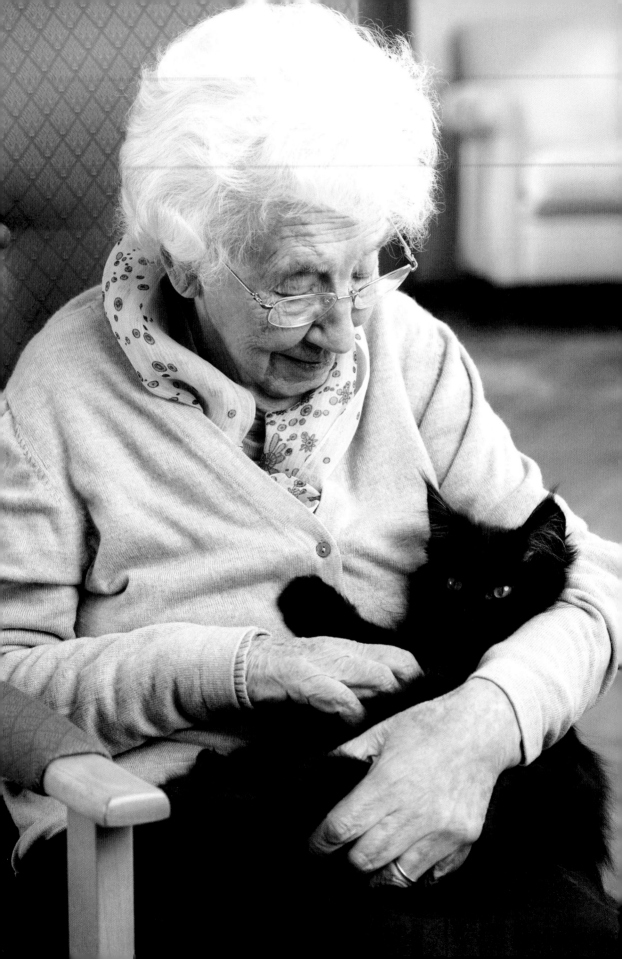

CHAPTER 5

Current Treatments for Alzheimer's Disease

The seven stages of Alzheimer's disease were described in the previous chapter. This chapter outlines what can be done at each stage to reduce risk for people with the disease or, if necessary, lessen or mitigate their symptoms. Some treatments require making changes in lifestyle habits (stages 1, 2, and 3), others involve the use of drugs (stages 4, 5, and 6). Stage 7 requires palliative care.

STAGE 1
(No Symptoms or Measurable Cognitive Impairment)

Primary prevention, an approach developed by Dr. Zaven Khachaturian that aims to delay the onset of the symptoms of Alzheimer's disease in people who are aging, is an important health-care strategy. If, as of now, we could delay the onset of

the symptoms of Alzheimer's disease by five years, 50 percent fewer people would be affected in less than a generation; a delay of ten years would lower the prevalence by 90 percent! Knowledge of the risk factors (Figure 22) and protective factors (Figure 23) involved in Alzheimer's disease makes this theoretically possible. These factors will be discussed in greater detail in Chapter 6.

All it would take is to change certain lifestyle habits and (or) treat the diseases that predispose people to Alzheimer's disease. However, we would have to be able to prove it prospectively, that is, using groups of volunteers with an equal risk at the beginning and who would agree to undergo randomly allocated treatment for extended periods (from five to seven years). This is entirely within the realm of the possible; the SystEur study, conducted by Dr. Françoise Forette in Paris, showed

RISK FACTORS FOR ALZHEIMER'S DISEASE

- Age
- Sex (female)
- Low education level
- Alcohol abuse
- High blood pressure
- Sugar diabetes

FIGURE 22

PROTECTIVE FACTORS FOR ALZHEIMER'S DISEASE

- High education level
- Moderate quantities of red wine
- Physical exercise
- Intellectual activities
- Social networks

FIGURE 23

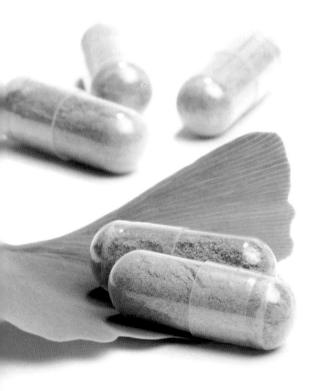

that stricter control of high blood pressure for five years cut in half the risk of dementia (especially that caused by Alzheimer's disease).

The GEM study, conducted by Dr. Steven DeKosky, in Pittsburgh, compared the effects of ginkgo biloba and a placebo for seven years, although his research was not able to show differences between the group that took the placebo and the group that took the ginkgo.

A team directed by Dr. Miia Kivipelto, in Helsinki, showed that it is possible to assess the risk factors for Alzheimer's disease around the age of fifty and thus to predict who will get the disease twenty years later: a total of 10 or 11 points were associated with a 7.4 percent risk and a total of 12 to 15 with a 16.4 percent risk (Figure 24). This assessment tool, the Dementia Risk Score, could be used in general medicine to inform people interested in finding out their risk level and motivated to act accordingly.

This kind of assessment could also be used in prospective studies to choose participants at comparable risk among interested volunteers. Including the APOE4 genotype in these risk factors would no doubt be necessary. We will come back to the genetic risk factors a little later in the book. Meanwhile, new tests such as measuring the levels of beta-amyloid in the cerebrospinal fluid (obtained via lumbar puncture) and positron emission tomography using ligands for beta-amyloid have been suggested (Weigand et al., 2011).

While awaiting the results of studies like these, which will very likely be carried out by major Alzheimer's disease research networks working together, people concerned about their health can also consult their family doctor to have their risk assessed, preferably before age sixty. In terms of society as a whole, initiatives to raise education levels and improve the quality of nutrition from a young age, like those proposed by the Lucie and André Chagnon Foundation, deserve support.

STAGE 2
(MILD SYMPTOMS WITH NO MEASURABLE COGNITIVE IMPAIRMENT)

Secondary prevention in people who do not have Alzheimer's disease but who are at higher risk may be possible if lifestyle habits associated with risk factors are modified, as described in the paragraph on treatments in stage 1.

Interestingly, studies in stage 2 can be completed more quickly than in stage 1, as shown by a study conducted by Dr. Bruno Vellas in Toulouse, comparing ginkgo biloba and a placebo for five years in stage 2, instead of seven years in stage 1. It must nonetheless be emphasized that the treatment administered in this study did not succeed in delaying the onset of Alzheimer's disease.

STAGE 3
(MILD SYMPTOMS WITH MEASURABLE COGNITIVE IMPAIRMENT BUT NO FUNCTIONAL DECLINE, OR MILD COGNITIVE DIFFICULTIES)

People in stage 3 have been the subject of much interest and research (reviewed by

DEMENTIA RISK SCORE

Factors	Criteria	Total points
AGE AT BEGINNING OF STUDY	Under 47	0
	47 to 53	3
	Over 53	4
EDUCATION LEVEL	10 years or more	0
	7 to 9 years	2
	0 to 6 years	3
SEX	Male	0
	Female	1
SYSTOLIC BLOOD PRESSURE	140 mm or less	0
	140 mm or more	2
BODY MASS INDEX	Less than 30 kg/m^2	0
	More than 30 kg/m^2	2
TOTAL CHOLESTEROL	Less than 6.5 mmol/L	0
	More than 6.5 mmol/L	2
PHYSICAL ACTIVITY	Active	0
	Inactive	1

FIGURE 24

Source : Kivipelto et coll., 2006

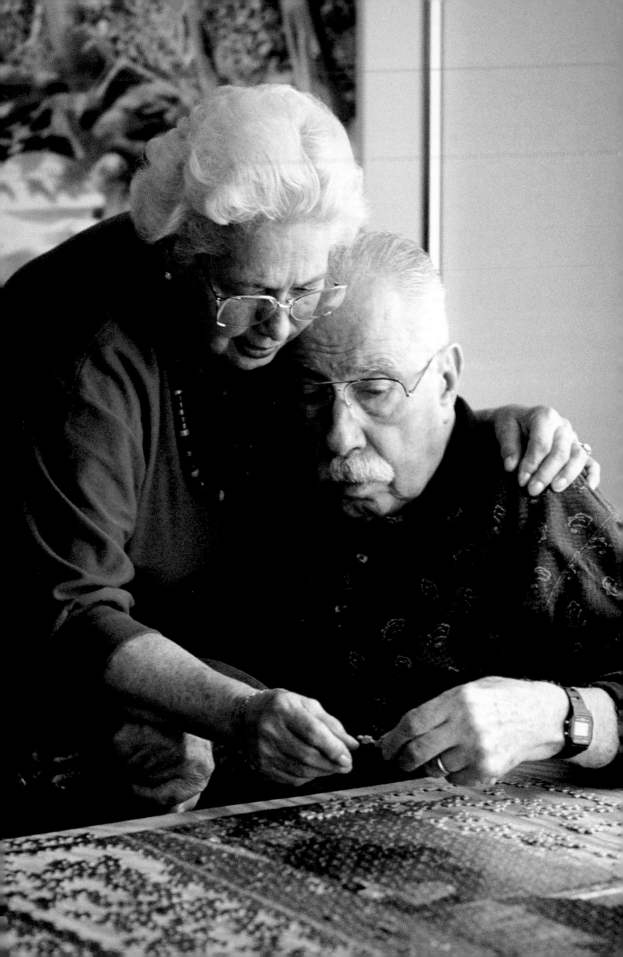

Gauthier et al., 2006). Several clinical trials comparing drugs with a placebo have been carried out, but without notable success in reducing symptoms (since these are mild, they are hard to reduce) or in delaying the progression to stage 4 (mild dementia).

We must remember that the causes of occasional forgetfulness in people in this stage may be very diverse and exist in combination: depression, professional exhaustion, sleep apnea, Vitamin B12 deficiency, drug abuse, malnutrition, hypothyroidism, etc. The appropriate treatment will thus depend on the causes of the symptoms.

If other possible causes of forgetfulness are eliminated, the presence of early-onset Alzheimer's disease can be confirmed (see Chapter 3 on diagnosis). The preventive advice outlined for stages 2 and 3 applies here as well, with closer follow-up and more rigorous treatment of vascular risk factors such as diabetes, obesity, and high cholesterol.

There are currently no "memory drugs" for people in stage 3, but cognitive training is being tested and the results obtained by Dr. Sylvie Belleville in Montreal are very encouraging.

A combination of cognitive training and supervised physical exercise, or "multi-domain treatment," is already being tested in Toulouse.

STAGE 4
(Mild Dementia)

Diagnosis of Alzheimer's disease in its mild stages must be discussed with the proxy and, if possible, with the person affected (see Chapter 3 on diagnosis). It may be useful to consult the Alzheimer's societies to learn about the disease. The patient's general health (and the caregiver's) must be assessed: it is essential to make sure their diet is adequate, that everything possible is done to enhance their vision and hearing, and that vascular risk factors are controlled (blood pressure, diabetes, auricular fibrillation). Drugs with negative effects on memory, especially those prescribed for bladder control, must be eliminated.

Symptoms of depression often occur and may require treatment with an antidepressant that affects levels of serotonin (citalopram, sertraline) or noradrenaline (venlafaxine). The therapeutic response is usually good and fast (between two and four weeks), using weaker doses than those prescribed for major depression in a younger person. The use of these drugs is usually halted after six to eight months, as people stop being aware of their illness and their mood improves over time. Potential (but rare) side effects include drowsiness or agitation, loss of libido, and trembling hands.

Cognitive changes — memory, language, spatial orientation, judgement — require the administration of drugs that act directly on the level of acetylcholine, the chemical transmitter produced by the brain that enables us to accumulate memories and engage in learning. There are currently three of these drugs in North America and Europe: donepezil, rivastigmine, and galantamine.

These drugs act by blocking one or two of the enzymes that break down the brain's acetylcholine: they are known as "cholinesterase inhibitors" (Figure 26). Figure 25 summarizes their main pharmacological properties.

Differences in the inhibition rates of one enzyme (acetylcholinesterase [AChE]) compared with the other (butyrylcholinesterase [BuChE]) and the activation of nicotinic receptors do not seem to be associated with significant variations in clinical effectiveness, at least not over a six- to twelve-month period. Current maximum doses are 10 mg/day of donepezil, 12 mg/day of rivastigmine orally, 9.4 mg/day via transdermal patch, and 24 mg/day of galantamine. The therapeutic response varies: in some people there is an obvious improvement in health in eight to twelve weeks, accompanied by a renewed interest in hobbies or daily tasks they had stopped doing. For other people (the majority) the situation is described by their families as stable, sometimes with a reduction in anxiety.

Symptoms may remain stable from one to two years, after which there will be a slow decline. Other patients, around 30 percent, experience a rapid decline in their intellectual faculties and ability to function, regardless of the drug used. These people are usually younger, female, and more highly educated

The possible side effects are listed in Figure 27 and vary little from one drug to another.

Fortunately, these side effects are largely avoided by taking the drug in the morning at breakfast, in gradually increasing doses. With the rivastigmine transdermal patch, many of these side effects are avoided, as the drug does not pass through the stomach. There can, however, be a mild skin reaction to the patch (redness and itching). An electrocardiogram is done before the patient begins to take these drugs if there is a recent history of unexplained fainting or a slow pulse (fewer than 60 beats a minute) with no obvious cause.

STAGES 5 AND 6
(MODERATE TO SEVERE DEMENTIA)

The therapeutic approach in these stages of the disease is similar to that in stage 4. It is never too late to try a drug that acts on

THE PHARMACOLOGICAL PROPERTIES OF CHOLINESTERASE INHIBITORS

	Donepezil	Rivastigmine	Galantamine
HALF-LIFE	70 to 80 hours	0.6 to 2 hours	7 to 8 hours
CURRENT MAXIMUM DOSES	10 mg/day	12 mg/day orally or 9.4 mg/day by patch	24 mg/day
DOSAGE	Once a day	Twice a day in capsules or every 24 hours by skin patch	Once a day
ENZYMES INHIBITED	AChE	AChE and BuChE	AChE
ACTION ON NICOTINIC RECEPTORS	+	+	+++

FIGURE 25

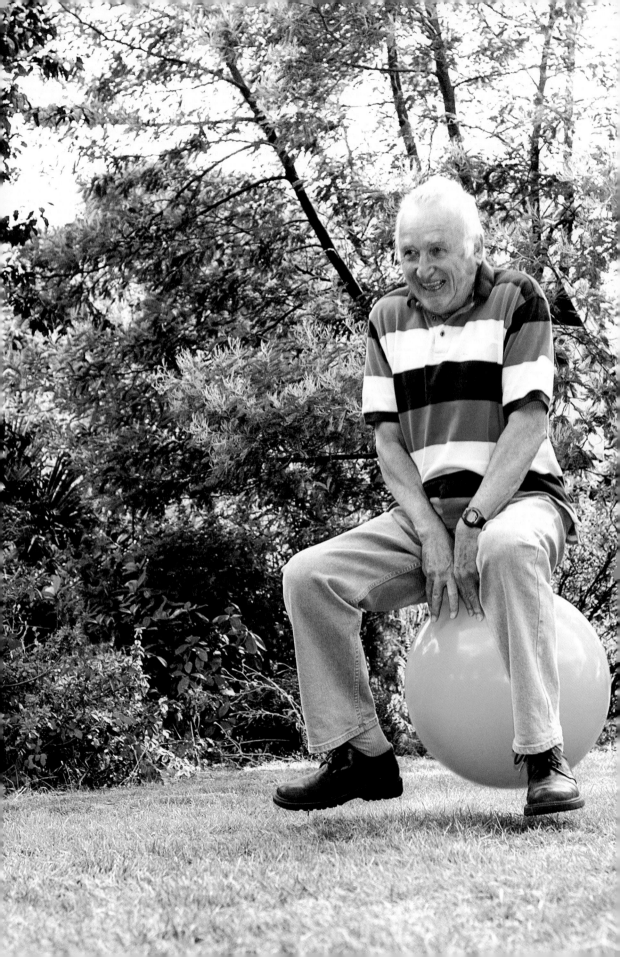

MODE OF ACTION OF THE THREE MAIN DRUGS USED TO TREAT ALZHEIMER'S DISEASE

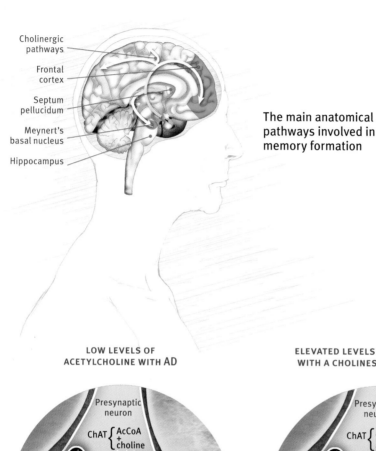

Cholinergic pathways
Frontal cortex
Septum pellucidum
Meynert's basal nucleus
Hippocampus

The main anatomical pathways involved in memory formation

LOW LEVELS OF ACETYLCHOLINE WITH AD

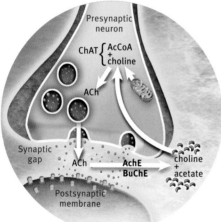

ELEVATED LEVELS OF ACETYLCHOLINE WITH A CHOLINESTERASE INHIBITOR

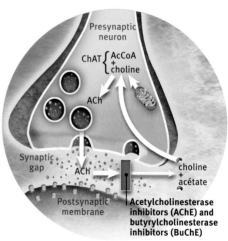

FIGURE 26

72

acetylcholine. Some studies suggest that the therapeutic effect is easier to observe in the moderate stages, because there are more symptoms that can be improved and the decline without treatment is faster and therefore more obvious.

To improve intellectual faculties — especially the ability to express oneself verbally — and decrease or prevent agitation or aggressiveness, memantine may be prescribed at this stage, along with acetylcholine inhibitors. This drug acts on glutamate receptors; glutamate is a chemical transmitter involved in several activities in the cerebral cortex, in the regions directly associated with memory and learning. It is taken orally in one or two doses, up to a maximum of 20 mg/day, and is excreted by the kidneys. Some people experience a better therapeutic result with a dose of 10 or 15 mg/day but become more disoriented or agitated at the maximum dose of 20 mg/day.

Dr. Oscar Lopez, in Pittsburgh, has shown that a treatment combining an acetylcholinesterase inhibitor with memantine, compared to treatment with an inhibitor alone or no inhibitor at all, delayed the need to transfer a person with the disease into a long-term care establishment. In other words, the progression of symptoms to the level seen in the advanced stages of Alzheimer's disease was delayed significantly by combining these two classes of drugs. Drugs with complementary effects are often combined in medical practice to treat, for example, high blood pressure, epilepsy, migraines, and diabetes.

Behavioural disorders appear or become more noticeable in stages 5 and 6 of Alzheimer's disease: apathy, aggressiveness, irritability, and restlessness. The most difficult problem for a caregiver is a person who does not sleep at night, does not recognize his or her house and family, and wants to

POTENTIAL SIDE EFFECTS OF ACETYLCHOLINESTERASE INHIBITORS

Gastro-intestinal effects	Nausea, vomiting, diarrhea
Cardiovascular effects	Bradycardia (slow heart rate), fainting
Neuromuscular effects	Cramps (especially in the legs)
Central effects	Insomnia, REM sleep behaviour disorder, increase in symptoms of depression or anxiety
Urinary effects	Frequent urge to urinate

FIGURE 27

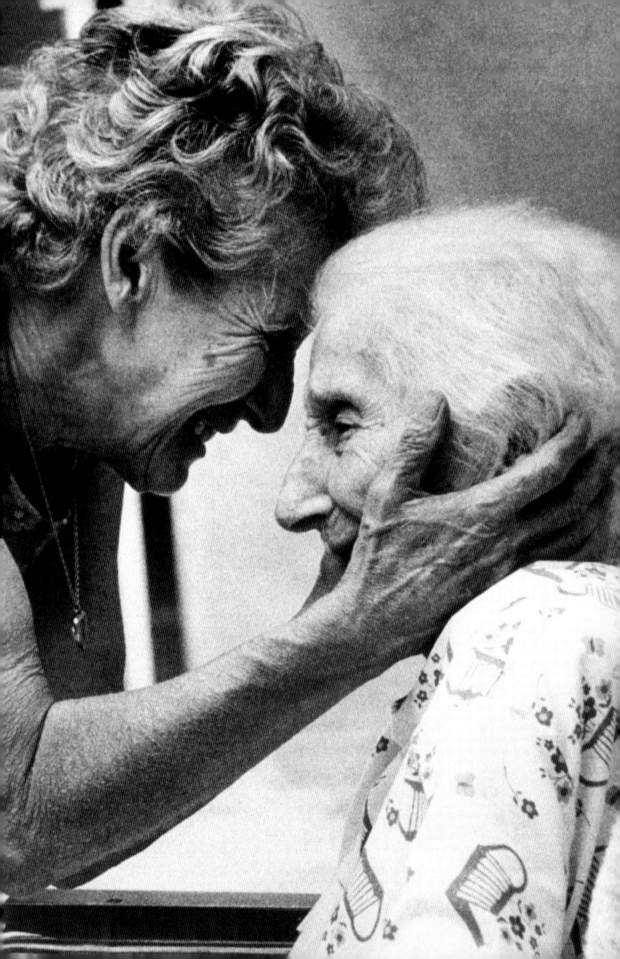

"go home." An antidepressant like trazodone at bedtime may sometimes help, but an antipsychotic drug such as risperidone must often be prescribed.

Since antipsychotic drugs slightly increase the risk of stroke or even death, they must be administered in small doses and only when there is no other option. The situation must be re-evaluated every three months, since behavioural symptoms tend to improve on their own after a period of time.

Other options include training offered to caregivers on behavioural disorders and on environmental changes they can make for example, more light, less noise, or changing bath time. Aromatherapy (especially the use of lavender) is becoming popular in England. Pets also seem to help Alzheimer's patients a good deal, especially cats, which of course, don't require as much attention from their owners.

Functional decline becomes more noticeable in each subsequent stage and people with Alzheimer's disease who live alone need more and more supervision to ensure their safety, which affects family, friends, neighbours, and community resources. People with Alzheimer's disease prefer to remain in their home as long as possible, but their safety and that of others must be taken into account.

People who live with a companion are luckier than those who live alone, but the caregiver does get very tired and needs to make use of all available resources: home help, assistance with bathing, meals on wheels, day programmes, and temporary breaks. Last but not least, the decision to place someone into a home must be discussed in stages 5 and 6, before the caregiver is totally exhausted.

STAGE 7
(VERY SEVERE TO END-STAGE DEMENTIA)

In our culture, the vast majority of people in this stage live in a care facility, but sometimes they can be kept at home with a great deal of help. Urinary and fecal incontinence occur and repeated falls require a wheelchair and then confinement to bed. Difficulty swallowing will eventually cause pneumonia.

An increasingly palliative approach to care is required at this stage of Alzheimer's disease, taking into account the wishes expressed by the patient when, in an earlier stage, he or she was still able to do so. More specifically, no further drugs are administered, except those required for comfort, such as acetaminophen for pain. This is not the time to start feeding the person artificially via intravenous, intranasal, or intragastric tubes, which neither increase longevity nor enhance quality of life.

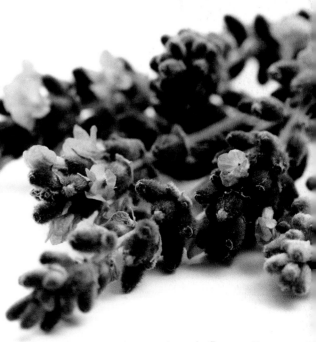

Lavender flowers. ↗

Care to be given in the event of pneumonia must be discussed with the legal representative: this may mean not transferring the patient to a hospital but rather providing palliative care with oxygen and morphine to allow the patient to die with dignity and without pain.

When the patient or the legal representative has openly expressed interest in a pathological examination of the brain for diagnostic purposes and research, a prior arrangement may be made with a brain bank, such as the Douglas Mental Health University Institute in Canada, or the brain banks of the Alzheimer's Disease Research Centres located all over the United States, at the Institut Pasteur and the Institut de Paris IV in France.

We will consider a little later, in Chapter 9, the major family decisions that have to be made in the key stages of the disease's progression. Some of these decisions are legal in nature, while others involve managing the drugs described in this chapter. No one should have to make these major decisions alone; these are decisions that will have significant legal, economic and familial ramifications if they were not considered at the right time by the patient and close family members.

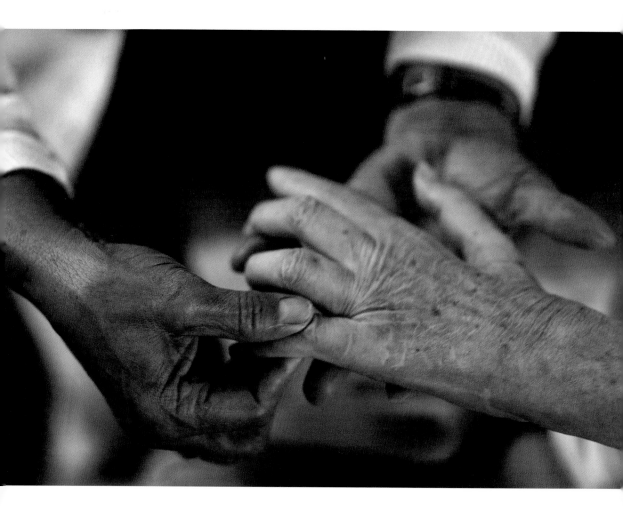

In Summary

Current Treatments for Alzheimer's Disease

Primary prevention (before any symptoms appear) offers hope for our society, since it takes into account risk and preventive factors. The effectiveness of secondary prevention (symptoms without impairment) will likely be easier to demonstrate through studies conducted in populations at known risk.

The interruption of the progression of mild cognitive disorders like Alzheimer's (the stage also called prodromal Alzheimer's disease or pre-dementia Alzheimer's) will be studied intensively in the coming years. For the moment, for people in the mild to moderate stages of dementia due to Alzheimer's disease, two classes of drugs can be prescribed that affect the activity of acetylcholine and glutamate neurotransmitters. The advanced stages of dementia require a palliative approach. At every stage of Alzheimer's disease, people must be able to retain their dignity and caregivers must receive all the help society can give them.

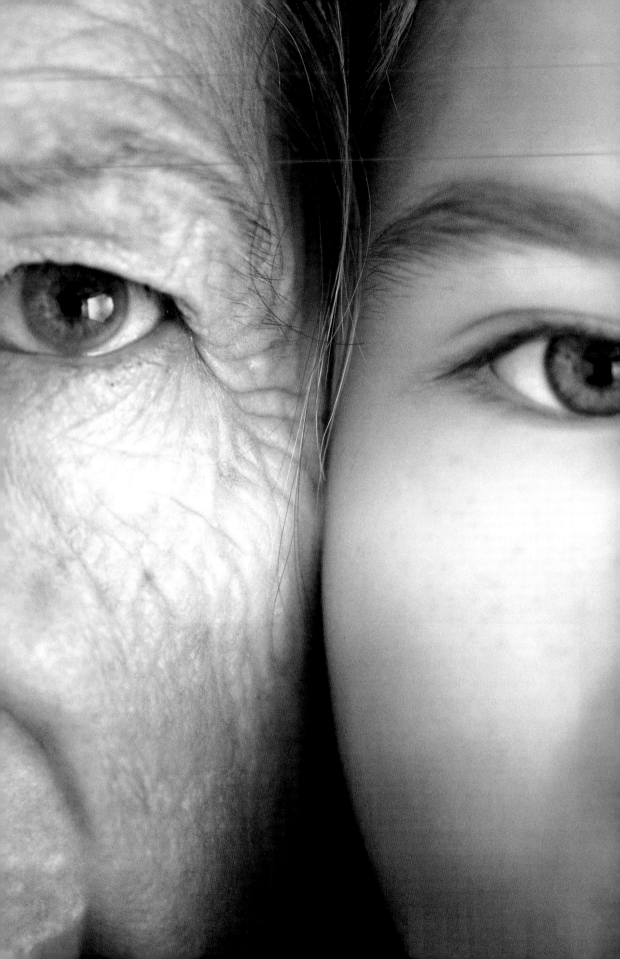

CHAPTER 6

One Hundred Years of Research into the Possible Cause of Alzheimer's Disease

Since Professor Alzheimer's original discovery over a hundred years ago, medical research has made dramatic progress, especially in the last twenty years. Systematic analysis of the pathology of the brain of Auguste Deter, the patient Alzheimer had monitored for several years, led to his discovery of a number of structural abnormalities still considered to be the classic markers of Alzheimer's pathology.

He described in great detail the disease's three main biological markers — now known more specifically as senile plaques, neurofibrillary tangles, and the massive loss of brain neurons. Even today, it is the presence of these classic markers that confirms a definite diagnosis of Alzheimer's disease during autopsy (Goedert and Spillantini, 2006).

In Alzheimer's time, these initial observations were greeted with a great deal of scepticism by his peers. We now know that these changes in the brain do not always result in dementia, since these abnormalities are sometimes found in the brains of normally aging subjects. These pathological changes may also be found along with other abnormalities in several rather rare kinds of dementia.

In the course of the hundred years since Alzheimer's discovery, many avenues of research have been explored to try to determine the probable causes of the disease. Among the variables that have most attracted researchers' attention, the age of the subjects is an obvious one, having been recognized over time as the main predisposing factor for the common form of the disease. Alzheimer's disease or dementia is very rarely seen in people under thirty.

In the decades following Alzheimer's initial observations, it was discovered that the large family of patients with the disease included a sub-group within whom the familial origin and transmission of the disease was extremely strong.

As a result, we now estimate at 5 percent the proportion of Alzheimer's patients with the "purely familial" type, while the remaining 95 percent are considered to be cases of sporadic Alzheimer's disease, more generally referred to as the common form of the disease. Precisely because of these preliminary observations, scientists in the middle of the twentieth century assumed that a large percentage of patients with Alzheimer's disease were likely victims of an environmental factor: for example, a virus, neurotoxin, bacterial infection, or perhaps a dietary disorder.

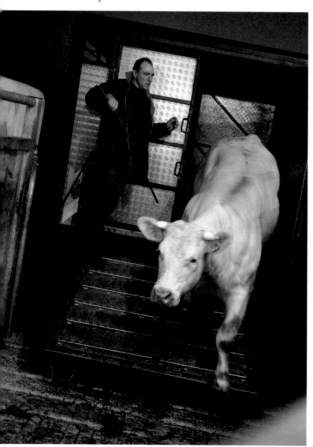

As we will see later in this chapter, researchers worldwide have indeed found scientific evidence to support a role for each of these risk factors in one kind of dementia or another, but not in Alzheimer's disease per se.

ENVIRONMENTAL FACTORS

This was the context that led the scientific community to focus its efforts on the environment during the first half of the twentieth century. In the 1950s, in the small town of Papua, New Guinea, a group of people was discovered that seemed to have spontaneously developed an environmental illness resembling a mixture of Parkinson's disease and Alzheimer's disease. This disease, later called "kuru," was especially concentrated in the small Fore tribe. It appeared to be transmitted from one individual to another by endocannibalism, a practice since banned, which involved eating some of a deceased person's organs as a gesture of respect (Lindenbaum, 2008). It was discovered that this disease, kuru, belonged to the large family of viral dementias related to Creutzfeldt-Jakob disease; in our western societies, the best-known of these is commonly called mad cow disease (see Figure 28).

We now know that kuru, like mad cow disease, is transmitted by a unique vector called a prion. This is a highly contagious disease for which there is no treatment and which, fortunately, has almost disappeared. These observations led scientists all over the world to examine nearly all known forms of viruses in the blood, as well as in the brains of people with Alzheimer's disease, but no causal link emerged from this research. Current international scientific consensus is that Alzheimer's disease is not viral in origin, even though some symptoms resemble those of kuru or Creutzfeldt-Jakob disease.

Once the viral hypothesis had been set aside, the first epidemiological studies suggesting that certain metals such as iron, copper, manganese, and even aluminum might play a role in the onset of Alzheimer's disease began to appear. For more than forty years, scientific evidence emerged from almost all over the world, timidly suggesting a possible role for iron and aluminum as risk factors in Alzheimer's disease. Unfortunately, for every study confirming this sort of link, an equal amount of contradictory evidence was obtained by various research teams, suggesting that these heavy metals played little or no part in the pathology of Alzheimer's disease.

It was only toward the middle of the 1990s, after a series of international scientific conferences, that researchers came to a global consensus. Scientific research based on the theory of a role for heavy metals, and aluminum in particular, in no way supported the conclusion that they played a possible role in Alzheimer's disease, neither in the onset of the disease nor in its progression. Occasionally publications that suggest a plausible link between these metals and Alzheimer's disease still appear today, but no irrefutable scientific evidence has yet been presented.

For all of these reasons, therefore, there is no need to get rid of aluminum pots, to stop eating food that comes in aluminum

CHARACTERISTICS OF A BRAIN WITH CREUTZFELDT-JAKOB DISEASE

Spongiform degeneration
Microscopically enlarged section of a brain showing typical changes caused by the Creutzfeldt-Jakob virus

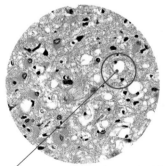

Holes can be seen (white bubbles), caused by the destructive effect of the virus on brain cells.

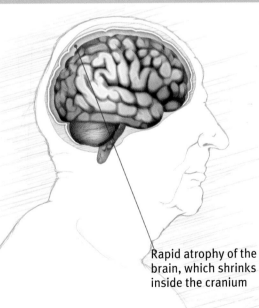

Rapid atrophy of the brain, which shrinks inside the cranium

FIGURE 28

cans, or to quit using antiperspirants (that's right! — their main ingredient being common aluminum salt).

Before we abandon the theory that a substance in the environment might be the source of Alzheimer's disease, mention must be made of the explosion in cases of severe dementia in Canada's Atlantic provinces in the middle of the 1980s. To everyone's surprise, a small epidemic of cases suddenly erupted, characterized by very serious cognitive impairment and memory lapses.

What the patients had in common was that they had all, in the previous hours and days, eaten freshly caught mussels from a neighbouring region. Upon enquiry, it was discovered that the mussels came from one specific fishing area, where an abnormal proliferation of a type of algae called diatoms was discovered. This strain of microscopic algae had contaminated the mussels caught along the Atlantic coast, releasing an extremely poisonous neurotoxin that could travel from the stomach to the brain in just a few hours. The toxin settled in the region of the brain called the hippocampus, whose main function is to coordinate the encoding and decoding of memories in human beings. The toxin had managed to damage the neurons responsible for memory and learning very seriously, causing symptoms similar to those of Alzheimer's disease (Doble, 1995).

Research has since led to the conclusion that common Alzheimer's disease is not caused by this kind of toxin and that there is no environmental toxin likely to cause similar damage. Although scientists have not completely ruled out the role of the environment as the only trigger for Alzheimer's disease, the most recent data clearly seem to indicate that what is at work in this neurodegenerative disease is instead something along the lines of a gene-environment combination.

GENETIC FACTORS

These research results thus lead us to consider the possible role that family history might play in the onset of the common or sporadic form of Alzheimer's disease. We have already mentioned that there is a purely genetic sub-group of the disease that represents about 5 percent of all known Alzheimer's cases (Figure 29). In these families, the disease is passed on from generation to generation in a "dominant" way; in other words, each child has one chance in two of getting it, going back centuries. It was realized in the 1960s that not only are there purely familial types of Alzheimer's disease transmitted over generations, but

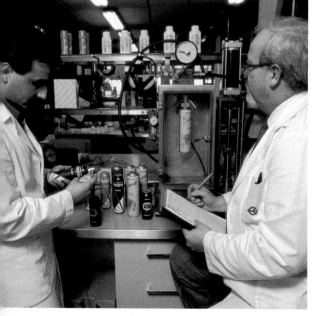

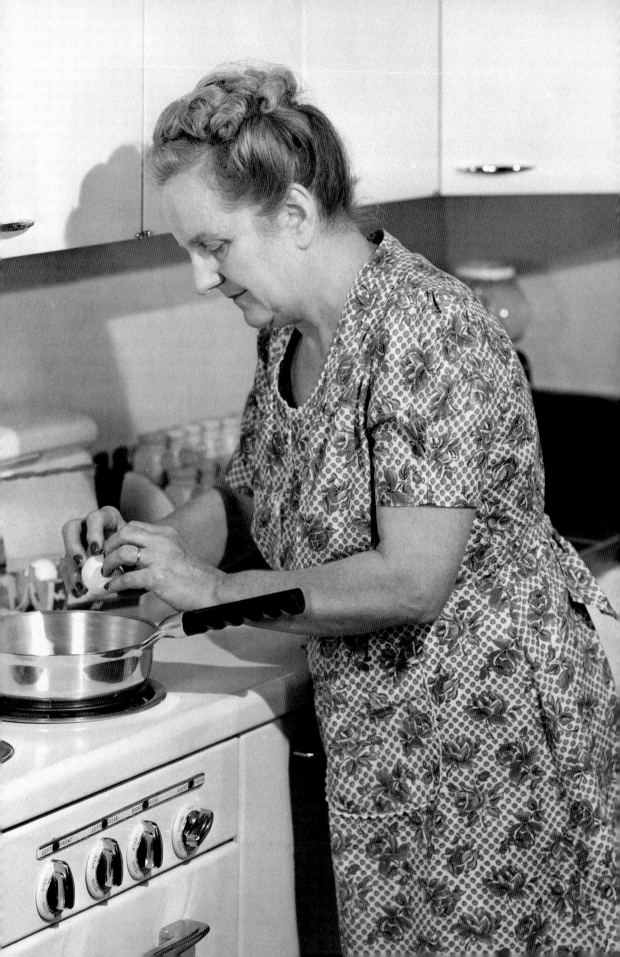

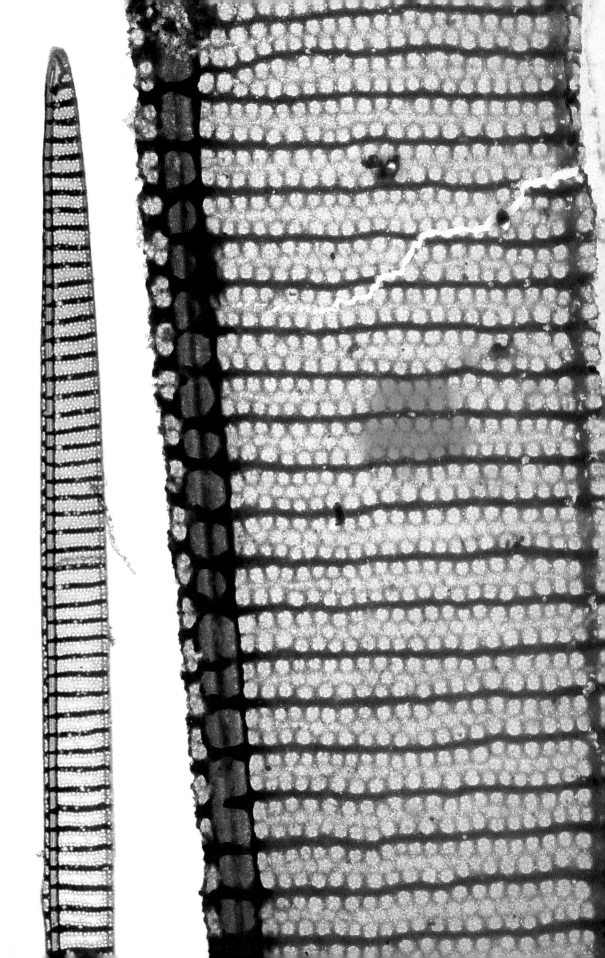

there seems to be a genetic predisposition that is also passed on to descendants. In fact, the idea is emerging that it may be the risk of developing the disease (and not the disease itself) that is passed on through generations in the common form of the disease. In this model of disease, it would be the combination of a genetic risk factor being passed on in the family and exposure to certain environmental trigger factors (think of obesity, high levels of cholesterol, etc.) that together could activate the pathological process eventually resulting in the onset of Alzheimer's disease. This etiological hypothesis for Alzheimer's disease is called the "ecogenetic hypothesis." Through studies of groups of identical and fraternal twins, researchers have managed to measure precisely how large a role genetics might play in the onset of common Alzheimer's disease.

Until the beginning of the 1990s, it was thought that the genetic contribution to Alzheimer's disease was somewhere between 25 and 80 percent of possible risk (Figure 29). Since 2000, this series of very large studies, in which thousands of pairs of twins participated, has made it possible to place the genetic risk at roughly 75 to 80 percent (Gatz et al., 2006). It is now clear that although we are talking about the common form, and not the familial form, of Alzheimer's disease, genetics still plays a paramount role. By studying the interaction of predisposing genetic factors and a high-risk environment, we will in a few years be better able to determine the specific causes of the various types of Alzheimer's disease. The scientific community is increasingly discussing the "diverse forms" of sporadic or common Alzheimer's disease.

To better understand the role of genetics and the environment in the development of Alzheimer's disease, we will individually examine the part that each of these two risk factors plays in the onset and spread of the disease in its various stages of impairment.

GENETICS AND THE COMMON FORM OF ALZHEIMER'S DISEASE

As we briefly saw earlier, Alzheimer's disease is subdivided into two major and very distinct types: the so-called "purely familial" forms, passed on from generation to generation and affecting 50 percent of the children, and the common form, which strikes more or less randomly in the population.

THE VARIOUS FORMS OF ALZHEIMER'S DISEASE

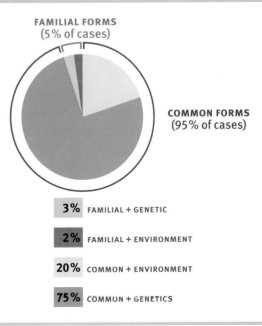

FAMILIAL FORMS
(5% of cases)

COMMON FORMS
(95% of cases)

3% FAMILIAL + GENETIC

2% FAMILIAL + ENVIRONMENT

20% COMMON + ENVIRONMENT

75% COMMON + GENETICS

FIGURE 29

↖ Two different-scaled views of the pseudo-nitzschia multi-series diatom, responsible for cases of dementia in Canada's eastern provinces in the mid-1980s.

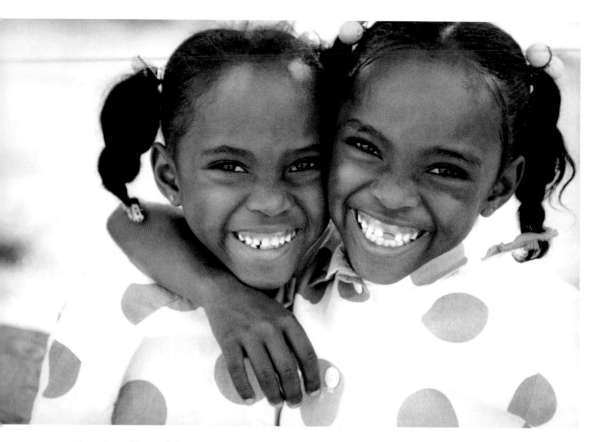

People affected by a purely familial form transmit the factor that causes the disease to 50 percent of the offspring in a given generation and there is no way stop or prevent the disease. These genetic familial forms are usually more aggressive and progress very rapidly. The early-onset familial form shows up in patients while they are still relatively young; in other words it usually appears between age thirty and fifty-five. There is also a familial form transmitted genetically that appears after age sixty-five. This form, which is somewhat more common in the population, usually accounts for no more than 3 to 4 percent of Alzheimer's cases in the West. In contrast to the early-onset familial form, scientists have not yet discovered the formal causes or genes that account for this sub-group of patients. However, a number of genetic risk factors similar to the risk factors usually associated with cardiovascular disease have been identified. We will examine these vascular factors in somewhat more detail in the section on the common form of Alzheimer's disease.

As for the early-onset familial form, in the past twenty years several groups of researchers, some of whom are working in Canada and France, have discovered three defective genes on chromosomes 1, 14, and 21 (St. George-Hyslop, 2000) (Figure 30). A patient born with one of these genetic abnormalities (a loss or gain of genetic material) cannot escape this time-bomb, for these genes really are responsible for causing the disease and are not just factors that increase risk. The discovery of these genetic causes of Alzheimer's disease in the course of the past two decades has led to a better understanding of the pathological and biological process at play in the development of the most extreme and aggressive form of Alzheimer's disease. On the other hand, it must be clearly understood that this fundamental scientific research applies only to patients with this form of the disease. The common form, also called "sporadic," progresses in a relatively different way and involves different genetic risk factors, compared with the aggressive, distinctively familial form.

Two distinct kinds of Alzheimer's disease can thus be identified with similar symptoms but several noteworthy differences. That said, it is clear that the way the brain reacts to the loss of neuronal cells associated with memory and learning is very similar in both forms of the disease. This observation makes it possible to devise new therapeutic approaches and new drugs that could not have been developed if not for discoveries made by studying patients with an aggressive familial form of the disease. By studying the biological processes in these familial forms, we have learned that the "senile plaques" described by Alzheimer are in fact the accumulated residue of a molecule we now call amyloid precursor protein, one of the proteins directly implicated in the early-onset and aggressive familial form. This protein, which through a rather complicated process breaks into fragments over time, gradually develops properties that are toxic for the aging brain (see Figure 31). The fragments of amyloid protein polymerize slowly, somewhat like polyurethane in plastic, accumulating for years and even decades in the brain. These masses usually form before the initial symptoms of Alzheimer's disease appear.

GENES INVOLVED IN THE FAMILIAL FORM OF ALZHEIMER'S DISEASE

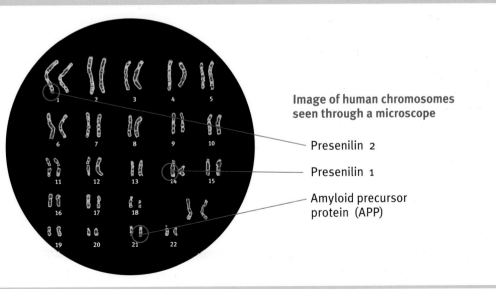

Image of human chromosomes seen through a microscope

Presenilin 2

Presenilin 1

Amyloid precursor protein (APP)

FIGURE 30

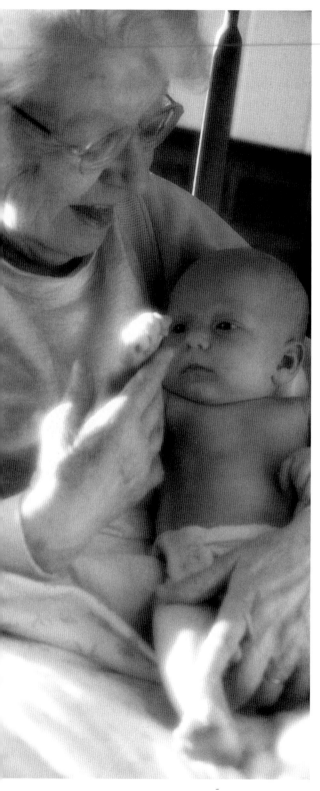

These observations suggest that a brain exposed to these toxic residues gradually binds the toxic molecules together in the shape of large compact clumps, which Professor Alzheimer described as more or less spherical senile plaques.

In recent years, researchers have also discovered that it is not so much the polymerization of this toxic protein that seems to pose a problem, but instead the overproduction of toxic amyloid fragments. This overproduction is thought to be the cause of death of the brain cells associated with the genetic abnormalities discovered in the three familial genes mentioned earlier, namely, the genes for amyloid precursor protein, presenilin 1, and presenilin 2 (Figure 32).

However, the precise mechanism through which the amyloid protein might poison brain cells remains rather vague. For a long time it was thought that the large amyloid spheres were the source of this toxicity. But recent scientific discoveries instead suggest that the brain's production of amyloid plaques is in fact a self-defence mechanism. In reality, the brain actually tries to isolate and immobilize the amyloid deposits so as to render them harmless for as long as possible.

This new way of interpreting the disease's pathophysiology rejects the idea that these much-discussed plaques are the main cause of the disease. They may instead be an effective defence mechanism aiming to neutralize the plaques' toxic potential.

Many research teams worldwide are now trying to determine whether amyloid protein, or some of its fragments, might not in fact be responsible for cell death. According to this hypothesis, the amyloid spheres scattered throughout the brains of patients with

Alzheimer's disease, as well as in those of elderly individuals who do not have any serious memory disorders, would not in themselves be responsible for cell death.

In Professor Alzheimer's preliminary report, there is a comment on the possible role of neurofibrillary tangles (NFTs). Large numbers of NFTs are found in virtually every part of the brains of Alzheimer patients. Recent genetic studies carried out in Europe and North America have resulted in the identification, beyond any doubt, of abnormalities in the tau protein, which, like amyloid protein, also has a tendency to polymerize and form long ribbons inside the cerebral neurons. These clumps of polymerized tau proteins are called neurofibrillary tangles. The normal function of tau is to maintain the integrity (the shape) of the neurons' intracellular skeleton structure. This structural component has been shown to collapse gradually over time as the tau protein is removed from the cytoarchitecture of the cell and becomes concentrated in the long ribbon-like structures called NFTs.

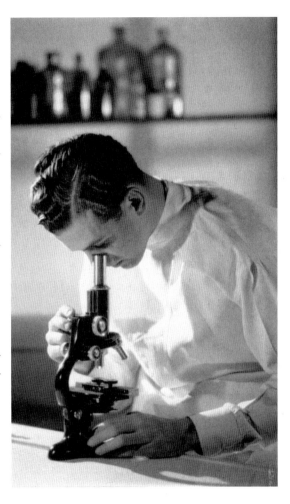

FORMATION OF AMYLOID PLAQUES

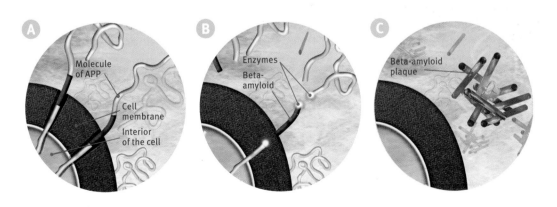

A Molecule of APP
Cell membrane
Interior of the cell

B Enzymes
Beta-amyloid

C Beta-amyloid plaque

FIGURE 31

PRESENILIN AND AMYLOID PRECURSOR PROTEIN (APP) IN THE CELL MEMBRANE

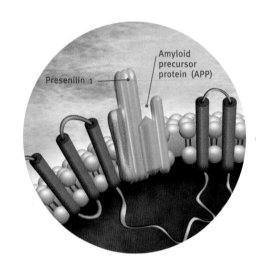

FIGURE 32

However, it should be noted that these familial forms of the disease, characterized by abnormalities in the tau protein gene, result in a type of dementia called fronto-temporal, as opposed to the common form of Alzheimer's disease. In fact, these are two diseases that are completely different from one another, even though there is some overlap in symptoms, including memory loss and a gradual deterioration in judgement. As with the early-onset forms of Alzheimer's disease, the genetic form of frontotemporal dementia is quite rare in the West.

This brings us to the largest group of people with Alzheimer's disease — the sporadic form, which represents more than 95 percent of all Alzheimer's cases reported worldwide. Up to now, scientists have not been able to identify a gene responsible for the common or sporadic form of Alzheimer's disease. However, our own research team and several others

DISINTEGRATION OF NEURONAL MICROTUBULES AND POLYMERIZATION OF PHOSPHORYLATED TAU PROTEIN

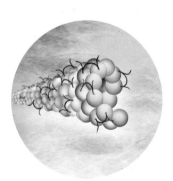
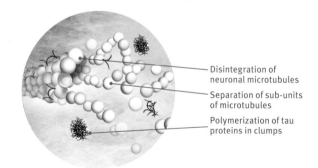

Intact microtubule (in its natural form)

Microtubule damaged by the disease's etiological process

FIGURE 33

THE TWENTY-FIVE MOST IMPORTANT GENES IDENTIFIED TO DATE AS RISK FACTORS IN ALZHEIMER'S DISEASE

Rank	Abbreviation	Name of gene	Associated pathologies
1	APOE E4	Apolipoprotein E	Risk of heart disease/cholesterol
2	APOJ	Apolipoprotein J	Risk of heart disease/cholesterol
3	PICALM	Phosphatidylinositol binding clathrin assembly protein	Cancer
4	EXOC3L2	Type 2 homologous protein associated with complex exocytosis type 3	Unknown
5	BIN1	Bridging integrator 1	Cancer/ Myopathic diseases
6	CR3	Complement receptor 1	Immunological diseases
7	LDLR-11	LDL receptor 11	Risk of heart disease/cholesterol
8	GWA-14Q32.13	Unknown	Unknown
9	TNK1	Tyrosine kinase (type 1)	Embryonic development
10	IL8	Interleukin 8	Inflammatory diseases
11	LDLR	LDL Receptor	Risk of heart disease/cholesterol
12	CST3	Cystatin C1	Risk of heart disease/cholesterol
13	hCG2039140	hCG2039140	Unknown
14	CHRNB2	Beta-2 nicotinic receptor	Epilepsy
15	SORCS1	Receptor for vacuolar protein triage type 10	Cancer/heart disease
16	TNF	Tumor necrosis factor	Inflammatory diseases/cancer
17	CCR2	Chemokine receptor-2	Inflammatory diseases
18	ACE	Angiotensin-converting enzyme	Heart disease/hypertension
19	DAPK1	Protein kinase associated with type I cell death	Cancer/embryonic development
20	GAB2	Type 2 protein related to peptide conjugate type 2 on the growth factor receptor	Cancer/embryonic development
21	TF	Transferrin	Blood cell formation
22	PCDH11X	Unknown	Unknown
23	MTHFR	Methylenetetrahydrofolate reductase	Cancer
24	LOC651924	Unknown	Unknown
25	OTC	Ornithine carbamoyltransferase	Multiple neurological deficits

FIGURE 34

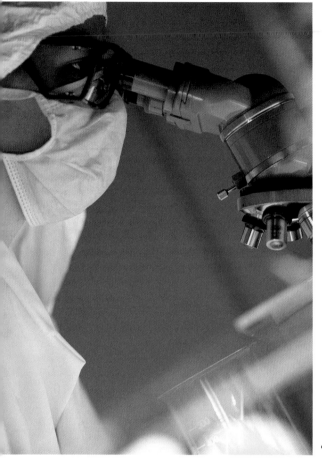

around the world have detected hundreds of different genes with genetic variations commonly found in North American and European populations (Figure 34). The presence of these genetic abnormalities significantly increases the risk of developing Alzheimer's disease. Some individuals have only one risk factor, while others have a combination of several.

Let's take a closer look at the four main genes that have been identified and linked to the common form of Alzheimer's disease. These genetic variations are now perceived to be the main players in determining the level of genetic risk for the disease.

The first gene, and without a doubt the most important to have been discovered, is the risk factor called apolipoprotein E type 4. First discovered by a team of researchers in North Carolina in patients with the familial form of the disease, this gene was independently identified in the same period by a Montreal team as being the main risk factor at play in the "common" form of Alzheimer's disease (Poirier et al., 1993). This discovery was

APOLIPOPROTEIN E: A CHOLESTEROL AND LIPID TRANSPORTER IN THE BRAIN

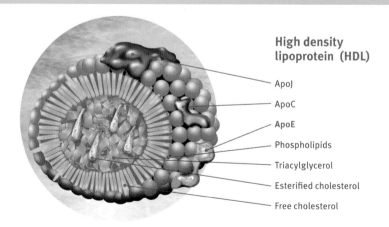

High density
lipoprotein (HDL)

ApoJ

ApoC

ApoE

Phospholipids

Triacylglycerol

Esterified cholesterol

Free cholesterol

FIGURE 35

to prove crucial in later years. Interestingly, the discovery was received with a certain amount of scepticism by the scientific community of the day. When the report was published, it was already well known that apolipoprotein E4 (APOE4) had an important role to play in the cardiovascular system in transporting and delivering blood cholesterol (Figure 35).

At the time, some researchers had trouble imagining how a blood cholesterol transporter could play such a predominant role in a disease that appeared to be almost exclusively limited to the brain. In the following months, however, the situation became clearer and the discovery finally made sense when it was learned that the brain contains more cholesterol than any other organ in the body. In subsequent years, our team discovered that the number of copies of the defective APOE4 gene that an individual inherits from both his parents at birth has a major impact on the age at which Alzheimer's disease appears and on its progression. Thus, the Montreal team accurately determined that people carrying two copies of APOE4 (one copy from each parent) have a greater than 90 percent risk of getting Alzheimer's disease. What's more, compared with people who have Alzheimer's disease but do not have the APOE4 gene, in people born with two copies of the APOE4 gene the disease usually appears between the ages of sixty-two and sixty-eight. In recent years, researchers have actually discovered that elderly people with mild cognitive impairment and who unfortunately have two copies of APOE4 will see their cognitive impairment worsen very quickly, causing the onset of Alzheimer's disease in their sixties, rather than at the common average age of seventy-five.

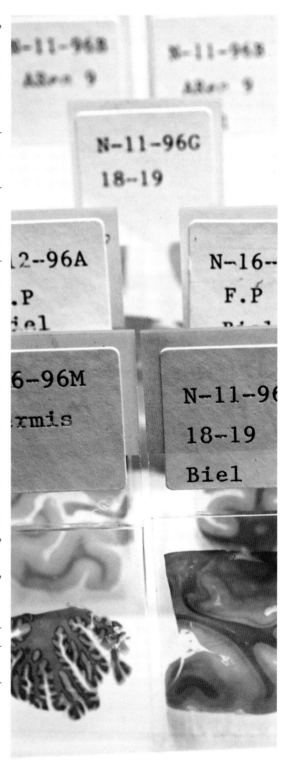

Brain slides prepared for examination. ⬀

In other words, while the apolipoprotein E4 gene is not the formal cause of the common form of Alzheimer's disease, it has a very major impact on the age at which the disease appears, on the speed with which it progresses, and, unfortunately, on the early onset of Alzheimer's disease symptoms (Leduc et al., 2010).

From a biological point of view, scientists have also discovered that the very nature of apolipoprotein E inherited from our parents affects the speed with which our brain will accumulate the senile plaques that are such a fundamental aspect of the pathology originally described by Alzheimer.

Among the genes that have been the focus of increased interest in recent years, it should be noted that in 2009 the biological partner of apolipoprotein E, called apolipoprotein J, officially became the second of these new risk factors for "sporadic" Alzheimer's disease (Lambert et al., 2009). This important discovery, made by a group of researchers at the Institut Pasteur in Lille, France, led to the identification of a third player that is just as important and is an integral part of our immune system. This gene, called "complement receptor 1" (CR1), enables the brain to better contain collateral damage caused by over-activation of the immune system in response to the damage to our brain cells brought about by the normal aging process or following damage caused by a neurodegenerative disease or a stroke.

Lastly, there is the butyrylcholinesterase gene, whose protein normally manages very effectively the production and degradation of certain neurotransmitters involved in memory and learning. It is known that, in most developed societies, approximately 4 percent of people are carriers of a genetic variation called "K," named in honour of Professor Werner Kalow, of the University of Toronto in Canada. However, over 30 percent of people with sporadic Alzheimer's disease appear to have this abnormal variant.

The presence of this abnormality speeds up the onset of Alzheimer's in people with mild cognitive impairment and, just as with APOE4, the presence of the K variant stimulates the accumulation of amyloid plaques in the brains of people with this abnormality. This variant also has a notable impact on how quickly the various forms of dementia, such as Alzheimer's, Lewy Body, and Parkinson's, progress. In short, although it is not a causal agent of the disease, the abnormal K variant of butyrylcholinesterase was shown to affect the transition to Alzheimer's disease and its progression.

Recently, our research team here in Montreal and other research groups in Europe and the United States have discovered that the K variant of butyrylcholinesterase has a serious negative effect on the therapeutic response to drugs commonly used to treat Alzheimer's disease. In other words, patients with the K variant respond only moderately to certain anti-dementia drugs, whereas patients who do not have the K variant have a markedly better therapeutic response when treated with other anti-dementia agents.

As was mentioned earlier, there are several hundred genes with genetic variations that have been very closely or distantly linked to the risk of getting Alzheimer's disease. But in contrast to APOJ, butyrylcholinesterase and complement receptor 1, the

Neurofibrillary tangles characteristic of Alzheimer's disease. ↗

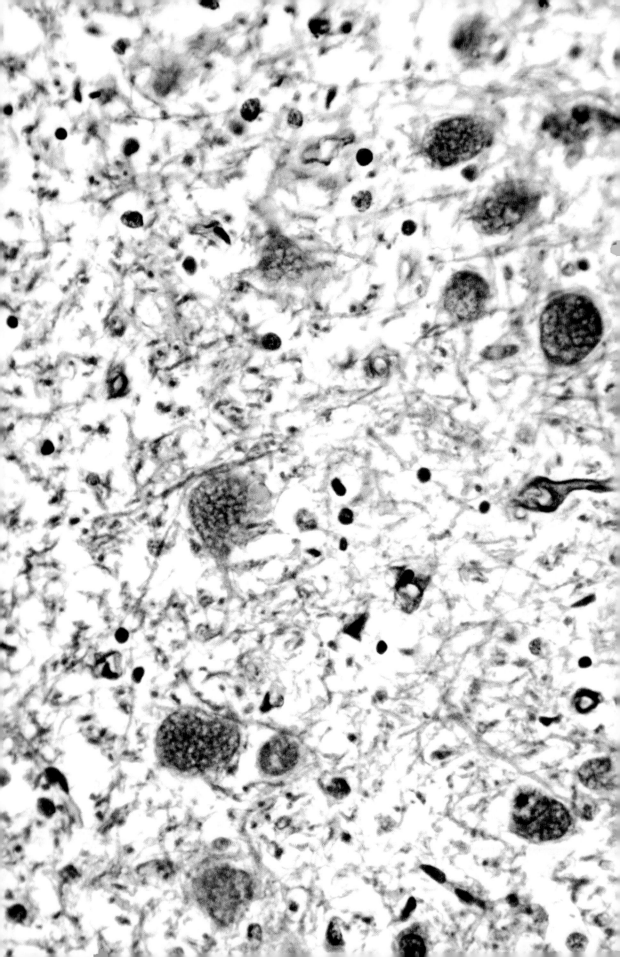

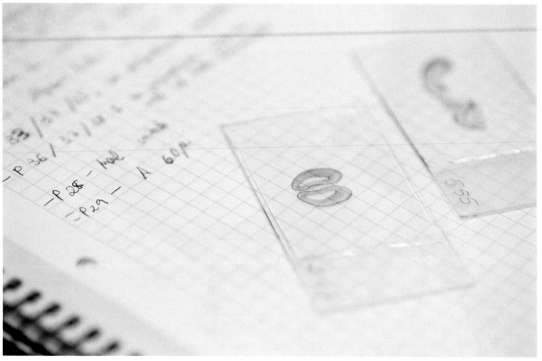

↗ Research slides close up.

connections between these defective genes and the common form of the disease has not been replicated convincingly in every human population studied worldwide — which suggests that a very large number of genetic risk factors are at work in every society. They occur in specific combinations that may be unique to particular ethnic groups or groups of people around the world.

Research work is underway in the largest genetics laboratories to combine genetic samples. The results of annual observations have been compiled during the last decade all over the world. The ultimate goal is to accumulate tens of thousands of samples so as to create the best genetic test possible; this could become the first genetic test able to determine, with a degree of accuracy hitherto unknown, the level of risk a person has at birth of developing Alzheimer's disease later in life.

ETHICAL CONSIDERATIONS AND GENETICS

At public lectures given by one or the other of the authors of this book over the years, we have often been asked about genetic tests for the familial and sporadic forms of Alzheimer's disease. In the case of genetic tests associated with the early-onset and aggressive familial forms, there are specialized centres in Canada, the United States, and Europe that can conduct genetic tests as part of long-term research projects. However, as with all genetic tests for fatal diseases, we strongly discourage having these tests performed without very close supervision of the patient by doctors who are specialists in the disease and a psychologist trained in genetic counselling. The situation would be totally different if we had an effective treatment that could stop the disease or even prevent it.

As for the sporadic form of the disease and testing for APOE, butyrylcholinesterase, APOJ, and complement receptor 1, we would discourage this even more strongly. We do not encourage the use of these tests outside of a controlled medical research environment. Even in this situation, it is highly likely that researchers will choose not to divulge the results of genetic tests to participants in a scientific study. The reasons are simple, and they are many. The first is of an ethical nature: the results of a biological test cannot be divulged if the test is not at least 99 percent accurate. But, as we saw earlier with APOE4, where carriers of a double copy of APOE4 have a risk in the neighbourhood of 90 percent, this means there is a margin of error of nearly 10 percent in the diagnosis of Alzheimer's disease. This situation also applies to biological tests measuring the levels of brain amyloids and of circulating tau protein. While the first scientific results are very encouraging on the diagnostic front, these biological markers cannot be used in everyday medical practice as long as the specificity and accuracy of the tests in large groups of patients worldwide have not been completely validated.

The second ethical aspect has already been discussed: the lack of curative or preventive treatment for the disease. In simple terms, this would be somewhat like condemning an innocent person to death without his being able to escape his fate. The third argument against using genetic (or experimental biological) tests to diagnose Alzheimer's at the current time is a legal one. Existing laws in Canada and France, while offering some protection from discrimination, are not as effective and stringent as American federal and state laws concerning the use of genetic information by a third party. Obviously, not only must genetic information be rigorously protected from all forms of manipulation, but employers, insurers, and even governments must not use this information for purposes of discrimination, whether positive or negative. There has been some progress in this area in recent years in Europe, but Canada still has a long way to go.

For these reasons (and several others) therefore, we are formally opposed to the large-scale use of partial genetic tests in the context of Alzheimer's disease. The situation will very likely change in five or ten years, when drugs designed to treat distinct sub-groups of Alzheimer's patients become available. Until then, we hope to see significant progress made, with respect to both legislation and the reliability of genetic tests.

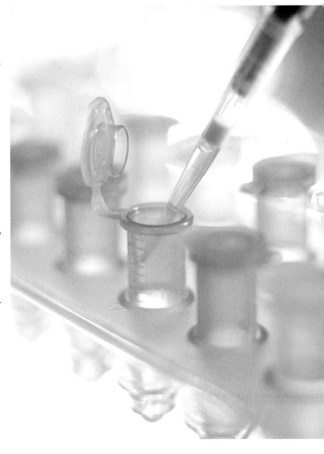

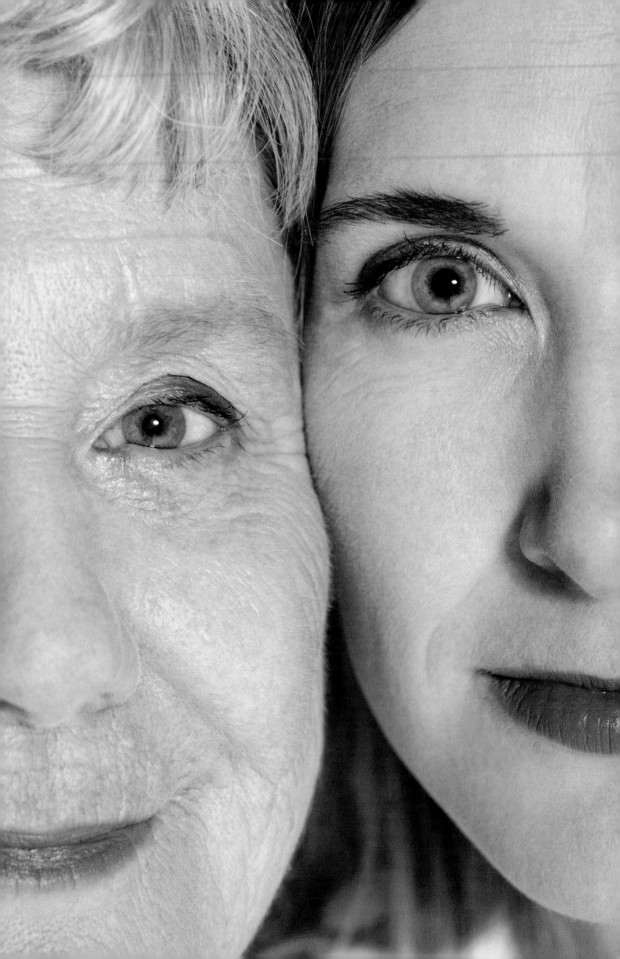

In Summary

One Hundred Years of Research Into the Possible Causes of Alzheimer's Disease

According to studies done on twins, the contribution of genetics to Alzheimer's disease is roughly 70 to 80 percent. In contrast to other forms of dementia, metals or viruses play no role in Alzheimer's disease etiology. There is an aggressive familial form of the disease that appears at an early age and for which three genes have been identified as responsible. The main gene at play in the common form of Alzheimer's disease is called apolipoprotein E. It is a key player in transporting cholesterol and lipids in the blood and brains of humans. Among the other genetic factors identified as being related to Alzheimer's disease are a significant number of proteins that play a role in regulating cholesterol and lipids.

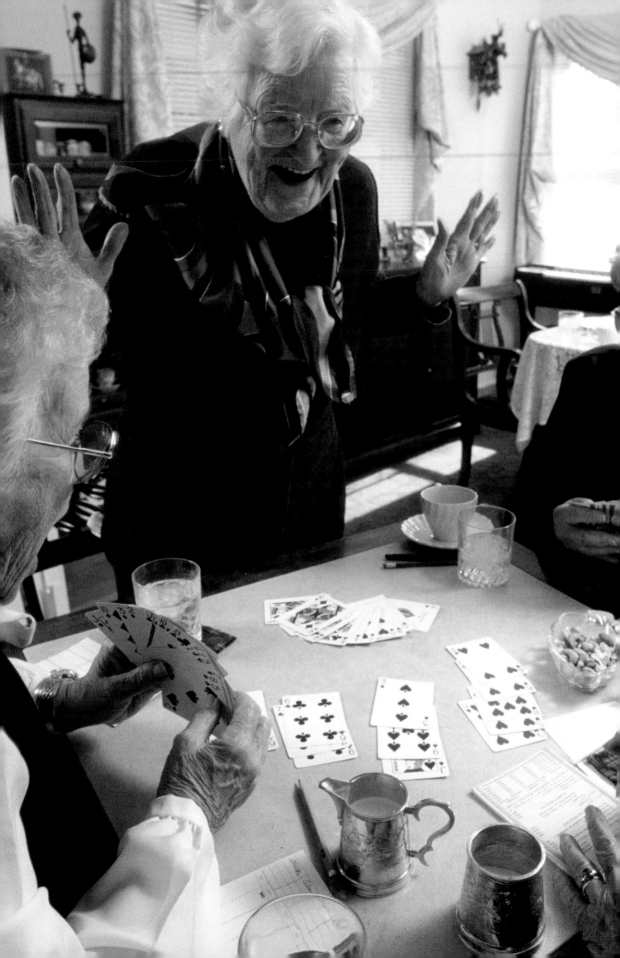

CHAPTER 7

Everyday Risk and Protective Factors

For several decades, researchers have successfully used epidemiological tools to identify, in large swathes of the human population, environmental or intrinsic factors specific to a given group and likely to increase or decrease the risk of developing Alzheimer's disease. The most important of these risk factors found in all the world's large societies is unquestionably the subject's age. Then comes what is generally called family history. For example, it has been known for more than thirty years that a person with a parent or grandparent who has or had Alzheimer's disease automatically has twice the risk of also getting the disease (Breitner and Folstein, 1984). The reason is very simple, as we have already seen: defective genes are directly responsible for the purely familial forms, while, for their part, genetic risk factors are directly responsible for the significant increase in the level of

risk of getting the common form of Alzheimer's disease. The large family of risk factors for Alzheimer's disease (Castellani et al., 2010) also includes:

- a family history of Down syndrome (mongolism)
- a personal history of untreated high blood pressure in one's forties or fifties
- a personal history of high blood cholesterol, also in one's forties or fifties
- a personal history of diabetes or metabolic syndrome
- a personal history of obesity with or without apnea
- fewer than twelve years of education
- a history of one or more head injuries

Several of these Alzheimer risk factors are also strongly associated with the risk of cardiovascular disease. In most cases, it appears that the use of drugs or specific diets can significantly reduce the risk associated with Alzheimer's disease.

In the opinion of a number of scientists, the very nature of these cardiovascular and Alzheimer's risk factors could partially explain the observed imbalance in the prevalence of the disease in men and women. As we saw earlier, two-thirds of people with Alzheimer's are women, while two-thirds of those with heart disease are men. Recent research suggests that, although several risk factors are associated with both diseases, the cardiovascular system is mainly affected in men in their forties and fifties, while women get through this cardiovascular risk period more easily, due in part to the presence of estrogen and related hormones. It follows that a second disease sensitive to the same risk factors awaits women between sixty-five and seventy-five. There are fewer men in this stage of life for the simple reason

that a significant portion of male subjects with risk factors have already died of heart disease in the preceding decades.

The good news is that using treatment tools commonly prescribed for heart disease, the risk factors for both these diseases can be proactively controlled and the role of cardiovascular risk factors in people likely to get Alzheimer's one day can be reduced. It is not just a question of taking drugs, but of measures as simple as exercising two or three times a week and eating a healthy diet low in animal fat, high in unsaturated fat like that found in fish, and high in fibre and vegetables, as in the Mediterranean diet. We will discuss later and in more detail protective factors and diets that have been validated by scientific research.

EDUCATION AND ALZHEIMER'S DISEASE

Education level seems to play a large role in the risk of developing Alzheimer's disease. People with twelve years or less have a higher risk of getting the disease (Katzman, 1993). Similarly, a higher level of education appears to have the effect of delaying the onset of memory disorders. As a result of a recent Swedish study on twins, in which one twin in each set was ill, we can now say with confidence that intellectual activity earlier in life seems to have an influence on the onset of the disease. Using data from the very large PAQUID study (Amieva et al., 2005), French researchers have also highlighted the influence of early intellectual activity in relation to cognitive aging after sixty-five. On the other hand, scientific data indicates that occupations in adulthood do not seem to have a determining effect

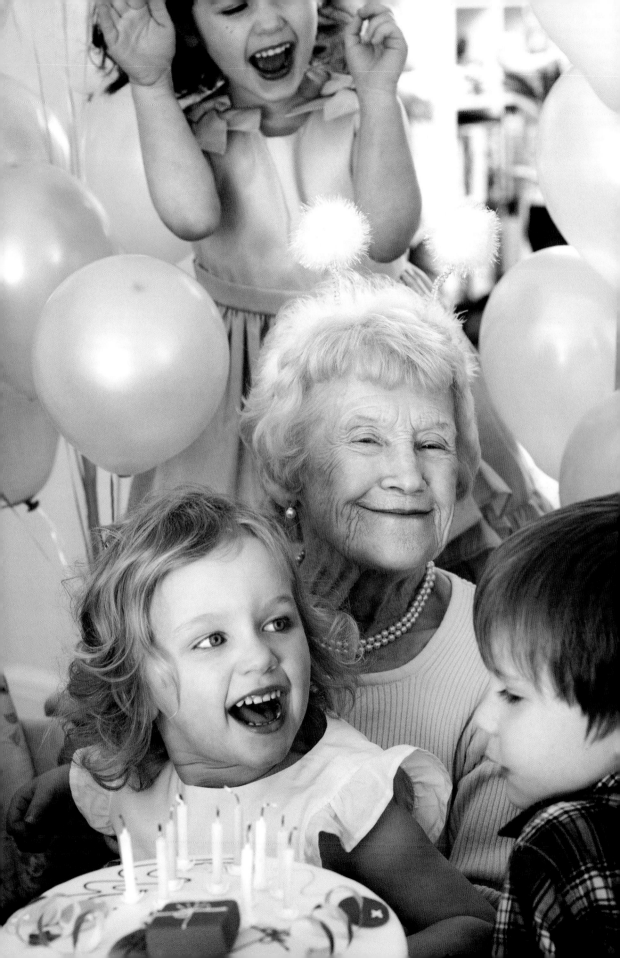

on the level of risk of developing Alzheimer's disease, compared with intellectual activities practiced in childhood and adolescence.

The explanation offered is that education continued for many years makes many demands on the brain and creates a kind of effective protection against the damaging effects of Alzheimer's disease. Such brains are better equipped to compensate for the damage caused by the neurodegenerative process; this enables them to continue functioning despite the damage they are undergoing. This explanation is known as the "synaptic reserves theory" (or the "cognitive reserve"), meaning that a brain stimulated by a cerebral activity maintained over the years creates an extended network of neural connections that better withstands the damage caused by normal or pathological aging.

In addition, in large-scale epidemiology studies around the world, several groups of researchers have examined the nature of the protective factors that might be likely to slow down the disease's progression and perhaps even prevent it.

Research on these protective factors in various western and eastern societies has led to the following realization: although a range of factors seem to provide a certain degree of protection, none of the factors identified to date seems to be able to slow down or stop Alzheimer's disease in someone who has already had it for some time.

In other words, several of these protective factors seem to have a cumulative effect if they are put into practice preventively before symptoms appear. In people already in the grip of the disease, they seem to have no effect.

Among the preventive factors that appear to be the most important, the following have been the subject of rigorous scientific investigations:

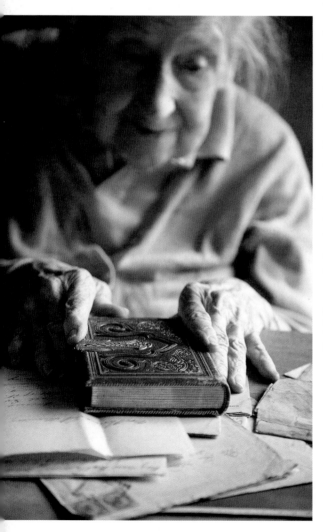

- more than twelve years of education
- low blood pressure medications
- blood cholesterol reducing medications (statins)
- antioxidants (Vitamin C, Vitamin E, ginkgo biloba)
- hormone therapy (estrogen)
- anti-inflammatory medications

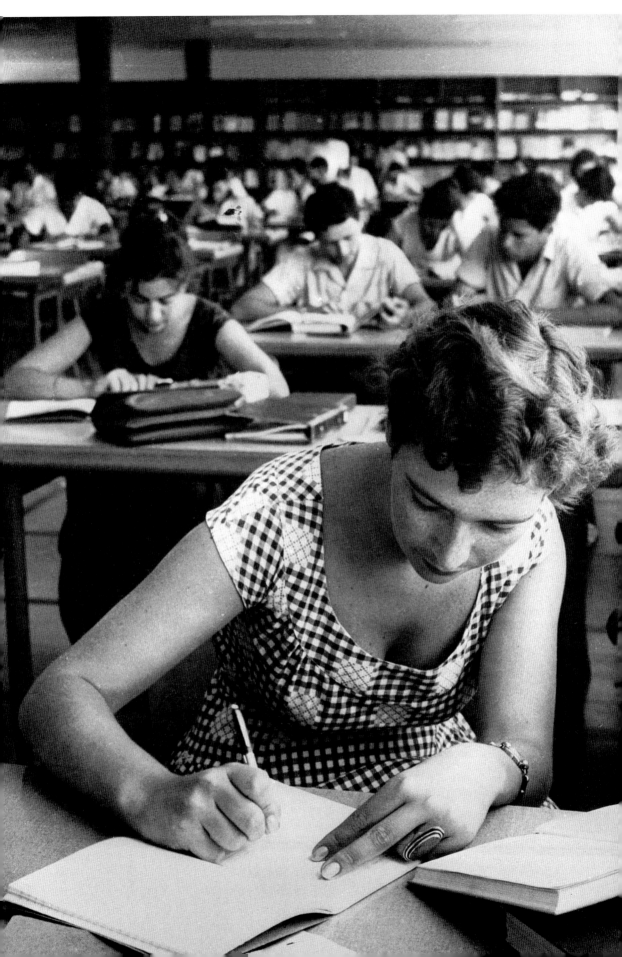

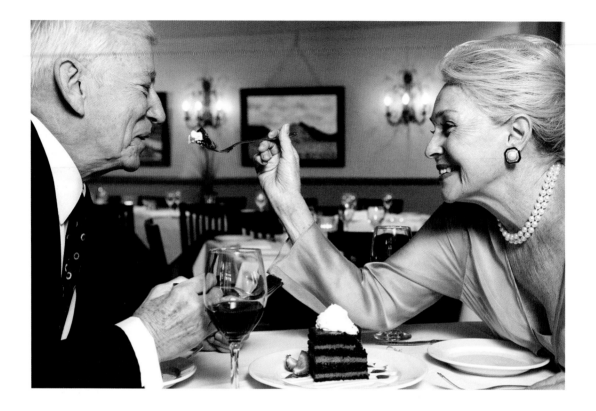

- red wine;
- a Mediterranean-type diet (low in red meat, high in poultry and fish, olive oil, vegetables, and grains)
- physical and intellectual exercises
- socializing

Obviously, these protective factors cannot be dissociated from the risk factors listed earlier. For every risk factor discussed up to now, it is possible that a combination of pharmacological treatments or various lifestyle habits may succeed in reducing or blocking the most significant negative effects caused by these factors. For example, if we look at the effects of antihypertensives or pharmacological agents that reduce blood cholesterol levels, it is clear that protection is intrinsically connected to the fact that better control of high blood pressure and blood cholesterol, in the years or decades preceding the probable onset of Alzheimer's disease, can reduce and even eliminate these two major risk factors. It should be noted that administering cholesterol-reducing agents or anti-hypertensives to patients who have been diagnosed with Alzheimer's disease does not seem to slow down in any significant way the progression of the disease, nor reduce its seriousness. In other words, the protective effect of these drugs applies mainly to those with high blood pressure or high blood cholesterol, and only if they are administered well before the onset of the first symptoms of Alzheimer's disease.

In the case of antioxidant agents, the situation is much clearer. Vitamin E, extracts of ginkgo biloba, Vitamin C, and ubiquinone do not in any way slow down the progression of the disease in those who have been diagnosed. The preventive administration of Vitamin E or extracts of ginkgo biloba in people at risk of getting Alzheimer's disease has no benefits in terms of memory retention or disease prevention. Across the board, the most solid scientific data in the field offer little hope: antioxidant therapy does not work, either before or after the onset of the disease.

For a long time, it was firmly believed that giving estrogen after menopause to women sixty years of age and older could guarantee a degree of protection against Alzheimer's disease. Epidemiological data still support the theory that there is a real benefit and a measurable positive effect with respect to memory and the risk of getting Alzheimer's disease in postmenopausal women taking estrogen. However, the fact cannot be ignored that large-scale studies carried out on postmenopausal women taking estrogen showed an increased risk of their developing certain types of cancer, including breast and colon cancers. What's more, administering estrogen to patients already diagnosed with Alzheimer's disease had no effect, positive or negative, on people participating in the study. What this means is that there is still no scientific proof to indicate that the progression of Alzheimer's disease is affected in one way or another by estrogen, whereas the use of this hormone in a pre-Alzheimer situation has effects that are far from negligible, especially in a long-term perspective, with preventive treatment administered for several years or even decades.

This brings us to the intriguing story of the role of anti-inflammatory medication in Alzheimer's disease. The first solid scientific evidence indicating that using anti-inflammatory drugs might be beneficial in Alzheimer's disease came from a group of researchers at Duke University in North Carolina (Breitner et al., 1994). During the 1990s, they managed to bring together a large group of sets of twins. The fundamental question being asked by the American researchers was the following: "What explains the fact that two identical twins, male or female (monozygotic), with exactly the same genetic heritage, begin to show signs of Alzheimer's disease five, ten, and even fifteen years apart?"

The only way to answer this question satisfactorily was to compare lifestyles and habits in identical twins. After having asked participants dozens and even hundreds of very personal questions, the researchers clearly saw that the twins who did not get Alzheimer's, or who got the disease much later, almost all had arthritis!

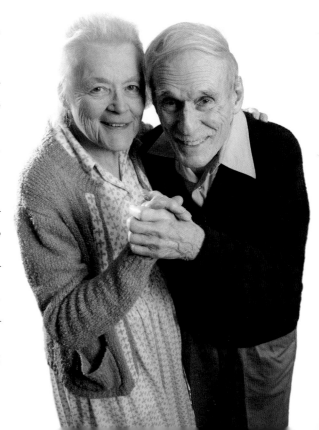

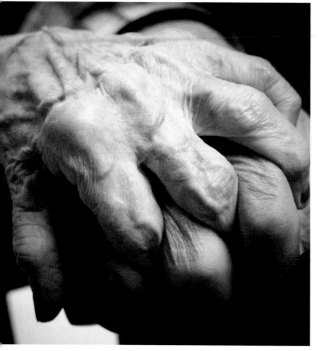

The researchers' first reflex was therefore to ask: "Does arthritis have an as yet unknown protective effect against Alzheimer's disease?" More likely, could the drugs commonly used to manage arthritis pain have an indirect beneficial effect on the progression of Alzheimer's disease (and on the risk of getting it)? Now, after ten years of research, it is quite clear that non-steroid anti-inflammatory drugs appear to have a measurable protective effect on people at risk before they show symptoms, whereas they have no beneficial effect in people who already have the disease.

These results as a whole suggest that the most promising window of opportunity if we hope to stop the disease is found in the years and even the decade before the first symptoms appear.

Fortunately, interesting ways to interfere with the progression of Alzheimer's disease have recently been discovered, in addition to the symptomatic drugs currently used to treat the disease. First and foremost, drinking red wine.

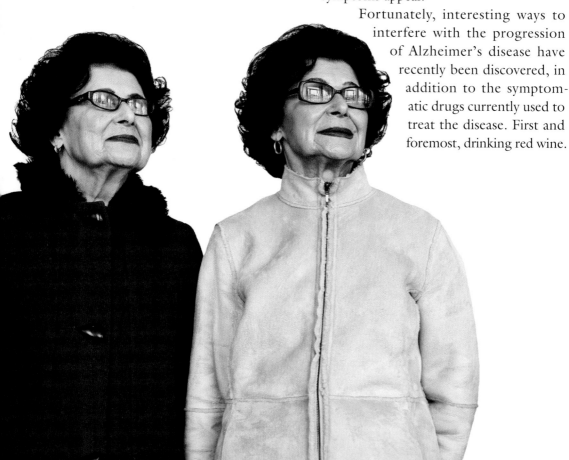

WHAT ABOUT RED WINE?

Studies of cardiovascular death rates show that the consumption of red wine follows an inverted U curve, meaning that the moderate consumption of wine has a beneficial effect, while abstinence has no effect and excessive consumption is harmful. Red wine must be consumed in moderation, regularly and with meals (from two to four glasses a day for men and one to two glasses per day for women). Red wine has many properties that keep atherosclerosis (blood vessel thickening) from developing, and recent studies suggest that it may offer some protection against Alzheimer's disease (Figure 36).

Note that red wine, in contrast to white, contains powerful antioxidants, known as polyphenols. These interfere effectively in the process of peroxidation (or oxidation) of fats we normally consume in meals. Among the best-known polyphenols in wine is resveratrol, which inhibits the oxidation of the cholesterol fraction contained in LDL lipoproteins (which is the same as the cholesterol normally carried in the blood), commonly called "bad cholesterol," as opposed to the good cholesterol found in HDLs.

Furthermore, red wine is a powerful blood vessel dilator. Dilation causes the blood vessels to begin to relax their smooth muscle coating, leading to vasodilation and thus an increase in the rate of blood flow. Red wine also keeps blood platelets from clumping in that it inhibits the formation of clots (thrombus) by hindering both the formation of clusters of platelets in the vessels and blood clotting. In a way, it acts as an antihypertensive agent. The first scientific study published in France on red wine, in 1997, linked the moderate and regular consumption of wine with a lower risk of getting Alzheimer's disease.

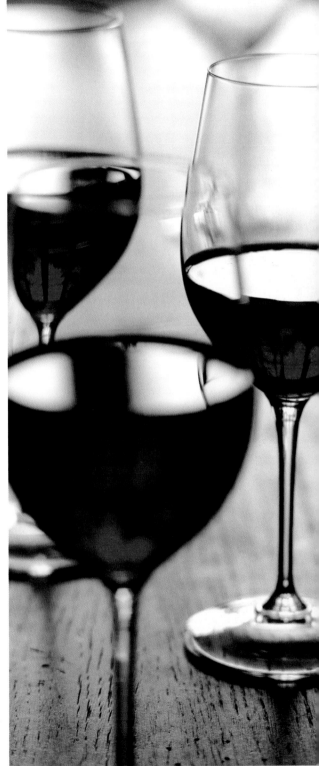

Two subsequent studies on individuals sixty-five or older have confirmed that drinking red wine — as opposed to drinking other alcoholic beverages like beer or white wine — is associated with a low risk of dementia, including Alzheimer's disease. Later, the Canadian Longitudinal Study on Aging, a major prospective analysis conducted in the Canadian population, determined that consuming red wine reduced the risk of Alzheimer's disease by nearly 50 percent. The questions we still have to examine in greater depth are: "What is the desirable quantity of red wine that has to be consumed for maximum effectiveness?" and "What wine is more effective for this purpose: French, Spanish, Italian, or New World?"

LIFESTYLES AND PERSONAL STRATEGIES

Recently obtained scientific results appear to indicate that certain non-pharmacological approaches may help prevent Alzheimer's disease, reduce some of its symptoms, and even alleviate worry in people who complain about the normal memory changes associated with aging.

PHYSICAL EXERCISE

Physical exercise, including fast walking, biking, swimming, or dancing, done three times a week, has a positive effect on the intellectual functioning of elderly people experiencing a slight intellectual or physical decline (people considered "frail"), but who do not have Alzheimer's disease. This has been demonstrated by comparing a group of people who exercised under supervision with a control group who did nothing in particular. A study in Seattle, in the United States (Larson et al., 2006), even showed that when physical exercise was maintained for six years, the symptoms of Alzheimer's disease were significantly delayed. On the other hand, it is important to be aware that jogging can cause some joints to age more rapidly and people may begin to experience chest pain if they start doing too much exercise without supervision. It is therefore wise to check with your family doctor first, and then to do the physical exercise of your choice at least three times a week, listening to your body so as not to increase the effects of aging on your joints.

INCREASING BLOOD FLOW

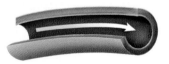

Normal blood flow

NORMAL
BLOOD VESSEL

DILATED
BLOOD VESSEL

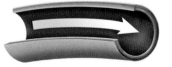

Increased blood flow caused by resveratrol

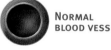

Resveratrol in red wine dilates the blood vessels

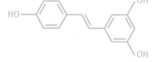

FIGURE 36

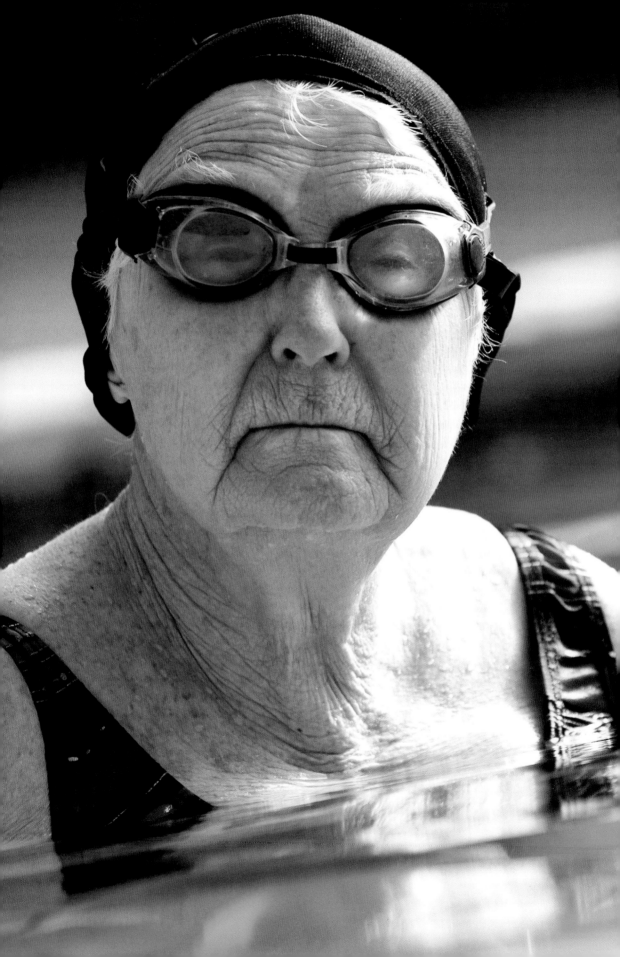

INTELLECTUAL EXERCISE

It has also been shown that intellectual training improves memory in people with mild cognitive impairment. The same is true of training in spatial orientation (through visuo-spatial tasks) or in decision-making (through management tasks). However this only leads to improvement in the specific area of training. Improvement in carrying out day-to-day activities has not yet been demonstrated as a result of these exercises, but Dr. Sherry Willis in Seattle was able to detect an effect on intellectual tests, as much as five years later, by comparing various groups of participants (Willis et al., 2006). Dr. Sylvie Belleville in Montreal has also observed a similar effect on memory tests, with the effect lasting at least a year (Belleville, 2008); a beneficial effect on brain function has even been shown using magnetic resonance imaging (Belleville, 2011). People who have already received a diagnosis of Alzheimer's disease do not seem to improve significantly, although a combination of disease-specific drugs and intellectual exercises seems to have a cumulative effect. It is therefore reasonable to advise everyone to keep their brain active doing something they like to do, preferably an activity that requires social interaction. There is no evidence that one intellectual activity is better than another, so the choice is quite varied: bridge, chess, crosswords, Sudoku, Facebook, Internet, and so on.

A HEALTHY AND NUTRITIOUS DIET

Epidemiological studies suggest that a Mediterranean-type diet rich in fish and olive oil, as well as fresh fruits and vegetables, reduces the effects of age on intellectual functioning (Frisardi et al., 2010). Recent clinical trials have shown that

If You Would Like to Participate in Research

If you have already been diagnosed as beginning to show signs of Alzheimer's disease, you can also participate in clinical research with or without drugs by getting in touch with one of the clinics in the Consortium of Canadian Centres for Clinical Cognitive Research, or with our research centre, whose contact information are found at the end of this book. You can also indicate in your health-care proxy in case of incapacity that you wish to participate in research on your disease, specifying that you understand there are risks if you try a new treatment, but in the knowledge that these risks will be monitored very closely by a research ethics committee and by the people you choose as your proxies.

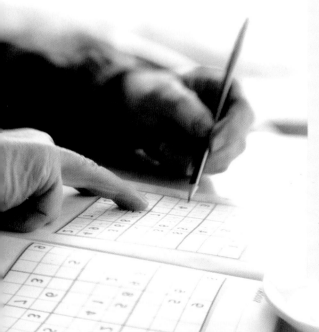

Omega-3 supplements lessen the symptoms of depression and improve some aspects of intellectual functioning. The Canadian Study of Health and Aging showed that people sixty-five and over who take vitamins have a reduced risk of intellectual decline after five years. On the other hand, too much of certain substances is harmful to health. For example, Vitamin E in the form of alpha-tocopherol increases the risk of death if taken in doses of more than 400 International Units (IU) per day. Too much folic acid (Vitamin B9) where there is no deficiency can be harmful to intellectual faculties. The best advice therefore seems to be not to take single-substance supplements unless you have a deficiency (for example, Vitamin B12), but instead to consume a varied diet incorporating the best elements of the Mediterranean diet. We will come back to this diet in Chapter 8.

A COMBINATION OF INTERVENTIONS

Several researchers in Canada, the United States, and France think that a combination of interventions (physical and intellectual exercise, a nutritious diet) may have a cumulative effect, lessen existing symptoms and perhaps delay the onset of Alzheimer's disease. A pilot study directed by Dr. Bruno Vellas in Toulouse is underway, involving people who are elderly and frail, but do not have Alzheimer's disease. In future, a large-scale study could be conducted in Canada and the United States. What is not certain, however, is whether it would be possible to restrict thousands of volunteers for such a study to a randomly allocated treatment (physical exercises alone, intellectual

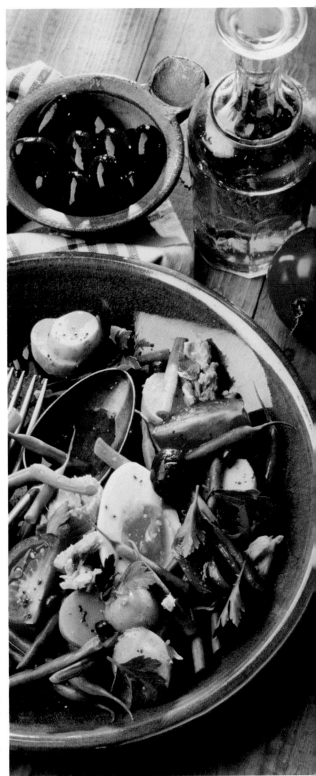

exercises alone, an enriched diet alone, or a combination of all three) for the five to seven years the study would last, since the temptation to do whatever it takes to remain healthy would be powerful.

HOW CAN PEOPLE TAKE PART IN MEDICAL RESEARCH?

We all hope to maintain or improve our memory. Research into mild cognitive impairment and Alzheimer's disease will thus have a positive impact on everyone, especially with respect to treatments not dependent on drugs, but rather on improving lifestyle habits. It is to be hoped that the protocols and exercises used in current studies will be made available to the public at large via the Internet and that the most useful exercises will thus become accessible to all of us.

For people who consider themselves to be at a higher risk of eventually developing Alzheimer's owing to their family history (essentially a first-degree relative — father, mother, brother, or sister), it will soon be possible to have a risk assessment done, using a scale that takes into account education level, weight, current age, blood pressure, cholesterol level, and physical exercise habits. Depending on each case, some of these people will be able to sign up as volunteers for large-scale studies on prevention that should begin in 2011 in Canada and France, as well as in the United States, once research funding is approved.

In Summary

Everyday Risk and Protective Factors

Although colossal amounts of money have been invested in medical research aiming to develop drugs to slow down or halt Alzheimer's disease, it is the approaches described as "non-pharmacological" that have suggested possible solutions, derived largely from cardiovascular medicine.

It has thus been discovered in large-scale studies (in which the results could be replicated) that doing moderate physical exercise several times a week perceptibly slows down the progression of the disease, and even delays it in individuals at risk but not yet affected. The same is true when a Mediterranean-style diet is adopted, low in red meat but high in white meat and fish, fruits, and vegetables. Even better, a combination of physical exercise and a Mediterranean diet appears to be strongly correlated with a delay in the onset of the first symptoms associated with Alzheimer's. Lastly, it has become equally obvious that healthy habits involving intellectual activity counteract in a slight but significant way the progression of the disease in people affected.

Each of these approaches, associated with behaviours rather than drugs, has measurable benefits, and even more so when they are combined.

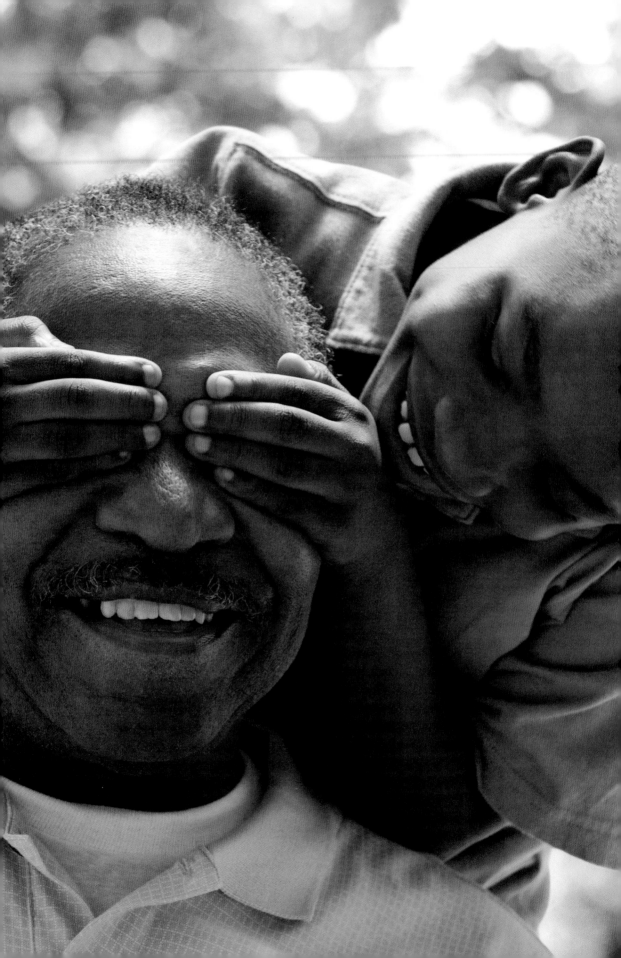

CHAPTER 8

The Shape of Things to Come, or Medical Research in the Years Ahead

In the last ten years, scientific research has enhanced our understanding of the fundamental mechanisms governing the onset and progression of Alzheimer's disease.

We are now aware of three intrinsic causes responsible for the early-onset and aggressive forms of purely familial Alzheimer's disease. Although this group of patients represents only a very small minority of cases, our understanding of the molecular mechanisms that are in play in these highly devastating forms of the disease has allowed us to recreate in a laboratory, in the brains of genetically modified mice, some of the fundamental components of Alzheimer's disease. Note that unlike common diseases such as cancer, diabetes, and stroke, we know of no other animal in nature that develops a neurodegenerative disease exactly like Alzheimer's in humans. This is partly why scientific progress in recent decades on Alzheimer's has been much slower than on diseases affecting peripheral organs like the liver or kidneys. Furthermore, the brain is without a doubt the most complex organ in our body and even today its functioning remains only very partially understood.

In this difficult research environment, scientists interested in understanding and shedding light on the fundamental causes of Alzheimer's disease have therefore had to resign themselves to using imperfect models recreated in a laboratory with tools that are at best an approximation of the symptoms and pathologies of a disease that affects human beings.

The obstacles researchers encounter in searching for new drugs are just as difficult to overcome and just as daunting in their complexity. Remember that the drugs available in pharmacies today are the result of scientific discoveries made in the mid-1980s, when accurately determining the chemical nature of the main control centres for memory and learning became possible. Shortly after this, researchers also managed to identify the regions of the brain affected by the degenerative process so typical of Alzheimer's disease. Once researchers had determined precisely the location and the seriousness of the loss of the chemical transmitters that control memory, pharmaceutical companies were able to get to work and develop active drugs that aim specifically to stimulate the brain cells still alive so they can work harder and longer.

These drugs, called "symptomatic" (symptom-reducing), are in fact chemical molecules (see Figure 37) whose primary goal is to prevent the destruction of the chemical transmitters that are already deficient in the brains of people with Alzheimer's disease. As their name indicates, these drugs act primarily on symptoms and do not have much effect on the normal progression of the disease. As a result, they do not prevent brain cells from dying and have only temporary effects, lasting from six to twenty-four months and varying greatly from one patient to another.

At first, researchers involved in testing these symptomatic drugs were convinced that we would only have to use them for a few years at most, pending the development of better drugs that would stop the disease from progressing. However, it soon became apparent that reducing symptoms is much easier than actually halting the disease. Since then, researchers worldwide have been taking their lead from discoveries made about the early-onset familial forms to develop new drugs that, it is hoped, will be able to attack the root of the problem, the cause of the progression of the common form of the disease. But here as well we have had to deal with many consecutive failures — the side effects of these new drugs outweighed the benefits, or the results were simply negative. Among the least serious side effects occasionally experienced are nausea, vomiting, or headaches.

Having chosen as the primary target the much-talked-about amyloid deposits (also called "senile plaques"), researchers have tried to use various strategies to block the production of the toxin, stimulate its degradation, and encourage its depolymerisation. Unfortunately, in every study undertaken to date, the results have been negative; that is, people given a placebo did just as well as patients receiving the active ingredient. These multiple failures have led some researchers, including the authors of this book, to seriously challenge the validity of the animal amyloid models being worked on, and especially the premises underlying the research, which suggest that what is abnormal in the early-onset and very aggressive familial forms of Alzheimer's dis-

MAIN SYMPTOMATIC CHOLINERGIC-TYPE DRUGS

Aricept
(DONEPEZIL)

Reminyl
(GALANTAMINE)

Exelon
(RIVASTIGMINE)

FIGURE 37

ease is also deficient in the everyday common form of the disease. In other words: "Is it possible that the early-onset familial form could be caused by deficiencies completely different from those that trigger the disease in its common form?" This would not be the first time in the annals of modern medicine. For example, Type 1 diabetes (the early-onset aggressive form) is caused by insulin deficiency, whereas Type 2 (the adult form) is not; as a result, treatment strategies now used to control the two forms of diabetes are different. The same is true of the early-onset form of juvenile Parkinson's disease, which is mostly familial in nature, while the common form generally appears around age sixty. Here also, the characteristics of the two forms are relatively different, as is the role played by genetics.

In addition, a foray into the field of anti-amyloid vaccines has also ended in failure, at least up to now. A small group of patients unable to tolerate the vaccine developed serious side effects, including encephalitis, some of which caused death.

It must be admitted that generally speaking, and not only in relation to vaccines, the field of therapeutic research devoted to Alzheimer's disease has recently gone through some rather bleak years. No new drug has received government approval since the launch of Ebixa, also called Namenda, in 2003. This drug, with its modest therapeutic effects, is only used in patients in the moderate or advanced stages, alone or in combination with one or another of the cholinesterase inhibitors.

Researchers have therefore gone back to the drawing board. Their primary objective: to extend the various fields of research so as to identify new therapeutic targets that

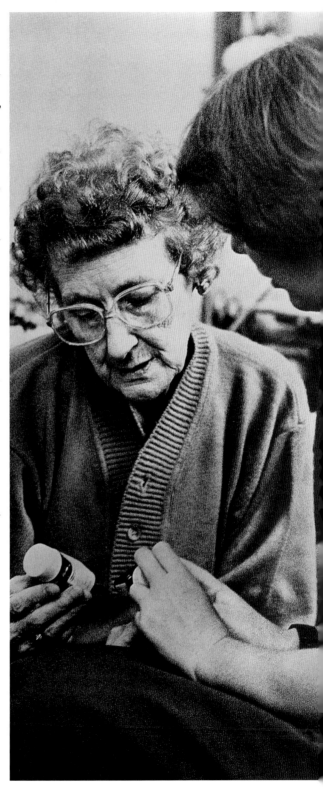

can be used to slow down, stop, and even prevent Alzheimer's disease. For about five years, new therapeutic approaches covering a whole range of molecular mechanisms have been in development. Let's look briefly at how they work.

Ebixa (Namenda)
(MEMANTINE HYDROCHLORIDE)

AMYLOIDS: PASSIVE IMMUNIZATION TRIALS

Having learned their lesson at considerable cost from the first tests of the anti-amyloid vaccine on human beings, the pharmaceutical industry has invested several hundred million dollars in developing second generation vaccines that would attack the amyloid deposits typical of Alzheimer's disease more directly. These new vaccines are currently under study. The most advanced version is being tested on four thousand patients in several countries around the world. This product has already been subjected to an entire battery of tests required by the various regulatory bodies in the countries concerned to ensure that the side effects and health risks are acceptable. Preliminary results, presented in 2008, while mildly positive, suggest that the vaccine will likely work most effectively in people who already have the particular genetic predisposition called apolipoprotein E3.

Still in the realm of attempts to reduce the production and accumulation of amyloids in the brains of people with Alzheimer's disease, several biotechnology companies are trying to develop pharmacological amyloid synthesis (production) inhibitors with much safer side-effect profiles than anything offered to date. At the same time, as more and more scientists challenge the focus on amyloids in the search for new drugs for Alzheimer's disease, a number of companies and universities have abandoned the "amyloid theory." For example, the Eli Lilly pharmaceutical company recently made it known that it is about to abandon this avenue of research after getting negative results with several of its experimental anti-amyloid drugs. From now on, therefore, researchers will concentrate on other therapeutic targets of interest. The following are a few promising examples.

DIMEBON: A SYMPTOMATIC AGENT OR A DISEASE STABILIZER?

Into this environment has come the first scientific data on a drug called Dimebon. This product, administered for the first time to treat Alzheimer's disease, has been used in Russia for more than thirty years as an antihistaminic drug, an active ingredient in fighting hay fever. Antihistamines are also commonly used to reduce the symptoms of the flu or a cold with a runny nose. The results of an initial study done in Russia indicate that this drug could also reduce

Dimebon

Alzheimer symptoms very significantly, right from the onset of the disease. However, recent North American and European studies have failed to replicate the benefits observed initially in the Russian population. Are we dealing with different populations, with some responding better to the drug than others? Is it a question of genetics, or is it simply a result of the fact that the latest studies used a sample much larger than the initial Russian study? The biochemical mechanisms that might give this pharmacological agent its therapeutic effectiveness are still rather murky, and preliminary results seem to indicate there could be both negative and positive effects associated with the use of this drug for long periods. To be continued....

NEW AND MORE POWERFUL SYMPTOMATIC DRUGS?

As we saw earlier, medications now sold in drugstores aim primarily to stimulate memory and promote learning or encoding of new information in our brains. These drugs have very few effects on the progression of the disease and the loss of brain cells.

That said, a new generation of memory-stimulating agents is under development in several pharmaceutical research centres. The most promising belong to the family of nicotinic agents (the same family as the nicotine used to stop smoking). These, combined with currently available drugs, could powerfully stimulate memory, make

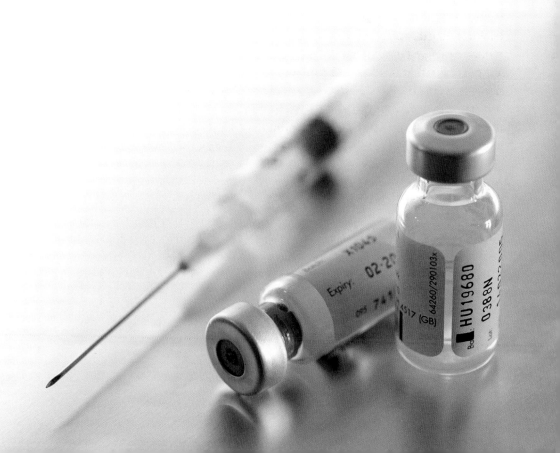

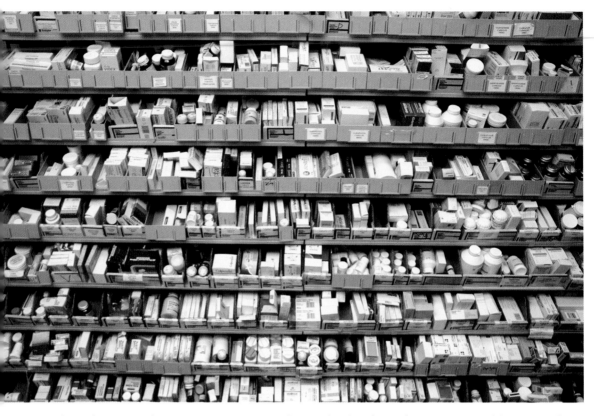

it easier to retrieve our recent memories and store them more effectively for a longer time. Several of these experimental drugs are now being tested in humans and should be on the market, if all goes well, within a few years. Obviously, as with all drugs, all side effects must pose absolutely no danger and the benefits of long-term use of these new drugs must significantly surpass those obtained with drugs now on the market. Nicotinic-type agents, in addition to actively stimulating the cells involved in memory and learning, can also stimulate neuronal cells to reconnect and help them survive in periods of intense biological stress. This is precisely what is generating so much interest in this new type of molecule, which seems to have a distinctive mode of action, but is perfectly complementary to drugs now used, in that

it stimulates the memory and increases the lifespan of neurons that are still alive, for a relatively long period.

Furthermore, some pharmaceutical and biotechnology companies have decided to develop symptomatic agents that are non-cholinergic (that is, they do not act on the neurotransmitter acetylcholine) and that might have properties that would considerably increase the memory capacity of people with Alzheimer's disease. Although most of these studies are only in the preliminary evaluation phase, encouraging results have been reported concerning molecules that stimulate serotonin receptors of type 6, as well as cerebral glutamate receptors — drugs in the memantine family (see the diagram on page 120). These molecules have been developed not to replace those commonly used now, but rather to complement their use in the various stages of Alzheimer's disease. For example, we know that at the outset of the disease, the effect of cholinergic agents in current use is somewhat weak compared with their benefits in the moderate and even severe stages of the disease. Being able, therefore, to enhance the beneficial effect on memory as soon as treatment begins, by combining two (or several) drugs, would be of considerable interest; this is what is known in medical jargon as "polytherapy." In addition, as the disease progresses, it becomes necessary to increase the effectiveness of the drugs to counteract the ongoing loss of brain cells. These various aspects of treatment and the adjustments required are currently being studied in several countries.

INCREASING THE LIFESPAN OF NEURONS: GROWTH FACTORS AND STEM CELLS

Not unlike the action of cholinergic agents, there is another biological approach that consists of reactivating the basic regeneration mechanisms latent in the brain from childhood. These mechanisms, which promote interconnections among neurons and sometimes even the division of brain cells, are called "growth factors." Practically speaking, these molecules behave somewhat like a foreman on a construction site. They give orders to the junior workers responsible for building new connections and new networks among the various regions of the brain (Figure 38). This makes it possible to stabilize the brain's "Internet network," known more formally as the neural network. It is precisely via these neural networks that the brain creates all the electrical connections required for thinking, memory,

movements, senses, etc. Growth factors play a crucial role in the foetal period, when these networks are developing, and during the first three years of life. In this decisive period the neural networks that connect the various regions of the brain for life are consolidated — hence the importance of the first three years of life.

These same growth factors make possible on one hand the creation of neural networks for storing memories, smells, visual images, and sounds, and on the other, all kinds of capabilities that give human beings the ability to move from place to place and interact with their immediate environment. Clearly, therefore, these crucial players in the development of connections among the various regions of the brain have a decisive role in shaping personality, attitudes, aptitudes, and up to a certain point, memory. Several biotechnology companies and a small number of pharmaceutical companies have developed very sophisticated ways of administering these growth factors to human beings. Unfortunately, the first series of studies, done in Sweden about ten years ago, failed, when very serious side effects causing severe pain in the arms and legs occurred.

The ways in which growth factors are administered has been refined since then. Four years ago, a California company succeeded in administering a concentrate of growth factors to a small group of people with Alzheimer's disease, using a nasal spray. The drug was able to measurably slow down the disease's progression. However, this research is in a very early phase, and there are still many stages to go through before these drugs are tested in large international studies in several hundred patients. The approach nonetheless remains highly innovative and promising.

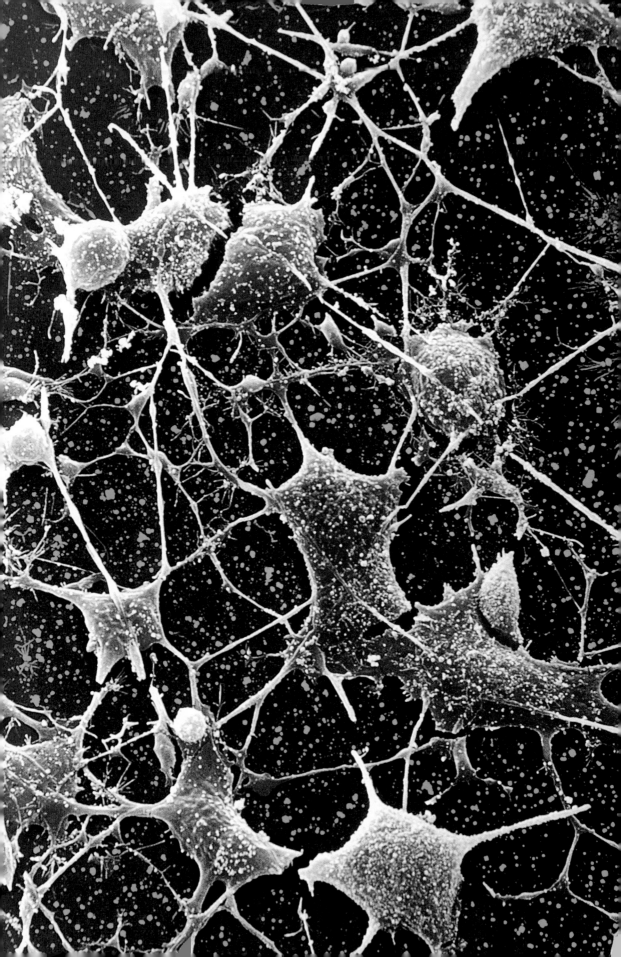

Studies derived from this approach are underway, using a unique mode of administration — a human cell genetically modified to secrete growth factors directly into the brain. The human growth factor gene has actually been successfully introduced into compatible human cells that have subsequently been transplanted directly into the brains of people with Alzheimer's disease in its mild or moderate stages. By means of this highly original approach, a source of continual production of growth factors (living cells) taken from the affected person can be inserted directly into the brain, using a long needle. If a person becomes his or her own cell donor, there is no possibility of rejection, since the immune system accepts the cells as its own.

To date, surgery remains the most difficult step to master. Since the 1990s, when the first surgical transplants of embryonic foetal cells were implanted in Parkinson's and Alzheimer's patients, surgery has resulted in a higher mortality rate. In Mexican and American studies, from 35 to 50 percent of patients died following surgery; since then, understandably, researchers and surgeons have been somewhat hesitant about using cell transplantation as a therapeutic method. There remains a long way to go before this cutting-edge technology is commonly used in hospitals.

The problematic situation with regard to brain surgery risk in elderly sick people also applies to what are called stem cells grown in a laboratory. These cells are generally taken from the patient who needs the transplant and are then subjected to intensive treatment with purified growth factors. This treatment outside the body has the effect of transforming stem cells into brain cells compatible with the person's brain.

In principle, there should be no rejec-

tion; it would thus become possible to replace dead cells with healthy new cells. Unfortunately, this does not reduce the risks of brain surgery, still as dangerous as ever. Similarly, the biological factors responsible for the death of brain cells in the Alzheimer's brain are still there and likely to attack the newly transplanted stem cells.

This is why we want to stress here that we — the two researchers and authors of this book — have many reservations about the media hype surrounding stem cells, which could, according to journalists, miraculously cure Huntington's chorea, Alzheimer's disease, Parkinson's disease, and even multiple sclerosis. In theory, these working hypotheses are attractive, but in practice we have very serious doubts, especially in the case of Alzheimer's disease. These diseases mainly strike older people who have a great deal of difficulty recovering from surgery, no matter what kind, but brain surgery in particular.

A GROWING NEURONAL CELL

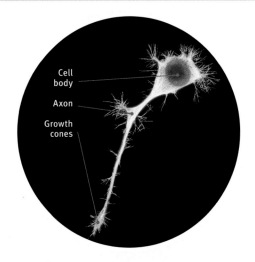

Cell body

Axon

Growth cones

EFFECT OF A GROWTH FACTOR ON THE EXTENSION OF NEURONAL PROJECTIONS (IN RED) IN A LIVING NEURON

FIGURE 38

↖ Image of neurons using a scanning electron microscope.

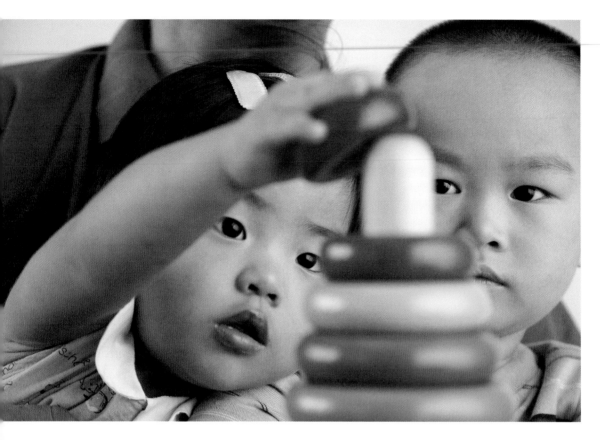

ANTIOXIDANTS: IS FURTHER RESEARCH WORTHWHILE?

The study of the use of antioxidants such as Vitamin E and Vitamin C in the treatment of Alzheimer's disease has long appealed to the public's imagination. It goes without saying that the fact these vitamins are easy to buy without a doctor's prescription makes them even more appealing. Old epidemiological studies suggested that the use of Vitamin E or Vitamin C could significantly delay the expected onset of Alzheimer's disease in high-risk populations. However, extremely well-controlled double-blind clinical studies (studies where neither the doctor nor the patient knows if they are using the active drug or a "sugar pill" placebo) have finally made it possible to eliminate once and for all the use of antioxidants like Vitamin E and ginkgo biloba in the prevention or treatment of Alzheimer's disease. These studies, which were very expensive to carry out, have clearly shown that, over a period of several years, these orally administered antioxidants have no beneficial effect whatsoever on the prevention of the disease or its progression over time. That said, it is not out of the question that other antioxidants that are more powerful or selective for the brain may be able to interfere in the degenerative process typical of Alzheimer's disease. We know, for example, that a large proportion of people who drink red wine see their risk of developing

Alzheimer's disease drop slightly. This has led researchers to analyze the various types of molecules commonly found in red wine (and not in white wine, beer, or other alcoholic drinks) and to purify those molecules with superior antioxidant properties. Among the thousands of components found in red wine, one particular molecule, resveratrol, seems to have the properties required to slow down the progression of Alzheimer's disease. Some biotechnology companies have purified resveratrol and are in the process of studying its use in small groups of people with Alzheimer's disease.

What is most interesting in this approach is no doubt the fact that resveratrol is a dietary supplement and not a drug. If resveratrol turned out to be sufficiently effective, it would be easier to obtain and it could be used without the person having to see a doctor.

WHAT ABOUT ESTROGEN FOR POSTMENOPAUSAL WOMEN?

We saw in an earlier chapter that while estrogen seems to have protective effects against Alzheimer's disease, according to prospective population studies, its use in postmenopausal women was associated with a higher risk of cancer. No woman should have to choose between cancer and Alzheimer's disease. Biotechnology and pharmaceutical companies have therefore developed chemical molecules resembling estrogen, but with a sufficiently

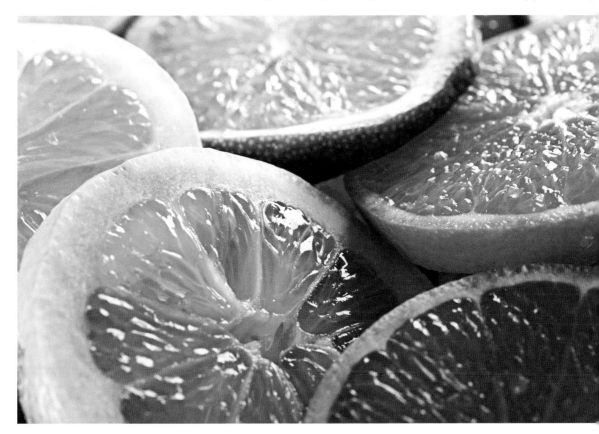

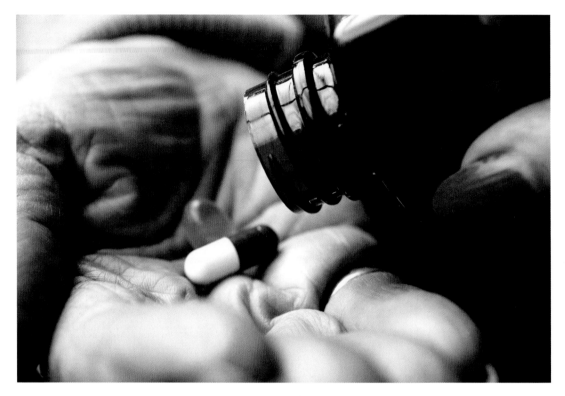

different molecular structure to eliminate the risks associated with breast and colon cancers.

One of the experimental drugs now being studied is raloxifene. This drug is already commonly used in treating osteoporosis and some forms of bone disease. By reducing the dose, researchers are trying to determine whether, in postmenopausal women, this drug could improve memory. We should know the results of these studies in a year or two.

IF DIABETES IS A RISK FACTOR, WHY NOT USE INSULIN?

Diabetes and metabolic syndrome (abdominal obesity and high blood pressure combined with high cholesterol) are now officially recognized risk factors for Alzheimer's

disease in people in their forties and fifties. Since these are clearly established risk factors, we might wonder if common treatments for these diseases, such as insulin and drugs that increase insulin sensitivity, might not have positive effects on the symptoms of Alzheimer's.

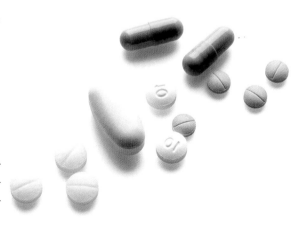

Based on preliminary observations, several studies have been set up in North America and in Europe to study the use of drugs in the glitazone family (Figure 39). These drugs are commonly used to treat Type 2 diabetes, whereas insulin is used to treat Type 1 diabetes, and sometimes Type 2. Very preliminary results presented last year at international conferences indicate that weak doses of insulin administered intranasally (as a spray) could have beneficial effects on memory and on the progression of the disease in a small group of precisely targeted patients.

Larger-scale studies with patients from various ethnic groups must now be undertaken. This will enable us to determine whether these drugs are beneficial for all Alzheimer's patients or only for a specific group.

On the other hand, two large-scale studies of rosiglitazone, commonly used in the treatment of Type 2 diabetes (adult-onset diabetes), have unfortunately failed to show results in people with mild and moderate forms of Alzheimer's disease. For the time being, we do not know if these studies will be repeated in people who do not yet have Alzheimer's, but who have genetic and familial antecedents. In that they are repeated, they would be aimed at prevention rather than at slowing down or halting the disease.

WHY NOT STIMULATE THE LAZY APOE GENE?

As we discussed in previous chapters, the apolipoprotein E4 gene is the most important genetic risk factor yet identified for the common form of Alzheimer's disease. Could this harmful gene not be targeted by one or more drugs in order to return it to normal biological functioning, which appears to be compromised in carriers of the E4 variant?

In fact, the field of research into drugs based on the genetic deficits associated with Alzheimer's disease has been booming for several years. Amyloids, which proved unsuccessful as a prototype for preliminary studies, have now been set aside in favour of new target genes. This is especially true of the APOE gene, which is currently the focus of research at three of the world's largest pharmaceutical companies.

Small-scale studies were conducted by the authors of this book several years ago, with very promising results. The first drugs designed to stimulate APOE production are expected to be tested in people in two or three years.

DRUGS USED TO TREAT DIABETES

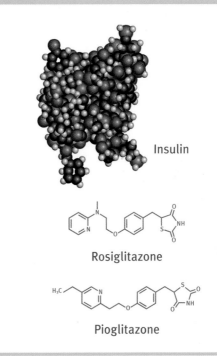

Insulin

Rosiglitazone

Pioglitazone

FIGURE 39

In university laboratories, where research is still at a very early stage, normal APOE genes have been successfully injected into the brains of mice using genetically modified viruses. The results have been dramatic, but transferring this technology from mice to human beings is likely to take several years, perhaps more than a decade. Human gene therapy, or the replacement of defective genes with normal genes, has unfortunately run up against many obstacles in the past fifteen years. The appearance of spontaneous cancers is certainly the most pernicious side effect we have encountered. While still in its infancy, this new science holds out great hope and scientific advances will eventually make it possible to overcome these harmful effects for the ultimate well-being of patients.

AND WHERE DOES PREVENTION FIT INTO ALL OF THIS?

In newspapers, in magazines, on the Internet, and even on television, many reports would have us believe that the best way to prevent Alzheimer's disease is to stay healthy by eating well and exercising ... as simple as that!

True, new trends clearly show that older people and baby boomers are making an effort to get more exercise than previous generations, and what's more, they eat better. Not only do they want to have healthier bodies, they are also absolutely determined to keep their minds healthy and sharp. Obviously, no one will be surprised to learn that there is great anxiety about brain diseases; this is especially so with regard to Alzheimer's disease, which often strikes the elderly,

who are more and more numerous in these early years of the twenty-first century. Sophisticated statistical studies have enabled us to accurately determine that if scientists could now delay the onset of Alzheimer's disease by five years, the actual number of people with Alzheimer's disease would be reduced by *almost half* in less than one generation. Better yet, if we succeeded in delaying Alzheimer's disease by roughly ten years, more than 90 percent of the number of people who now have Alzheimer's disease would be able to die of old age rather than from the disease. It is obvious therefore that the goal of delaying the onset of Alzheimer's disease looks much more promising than that of reversing the loss of brain cells in people who have already been diagnosed.

For about ten years, a number of researchers in the United States and Europe have been devising large-scale experimental studies. These studies have made it possible to evaluate harmless experimental drugs with enough potential for prevention to justify an enormous investment and several years of research. That said, most of the prevention studies carried out in recent years have had a somewhat qualified success, as the following explains.

Two distinct approaches have been used to identify the drugs most likely to delay the onset of Alzheimer's disease. The first approach targeted a group of people who were already experiencing memory disorders much more serious than are normally seen in healthy older people in stage 3, as described in Chapter 4. On the other hand, their cognitive impairment was in fact much less significant than that normally observed in

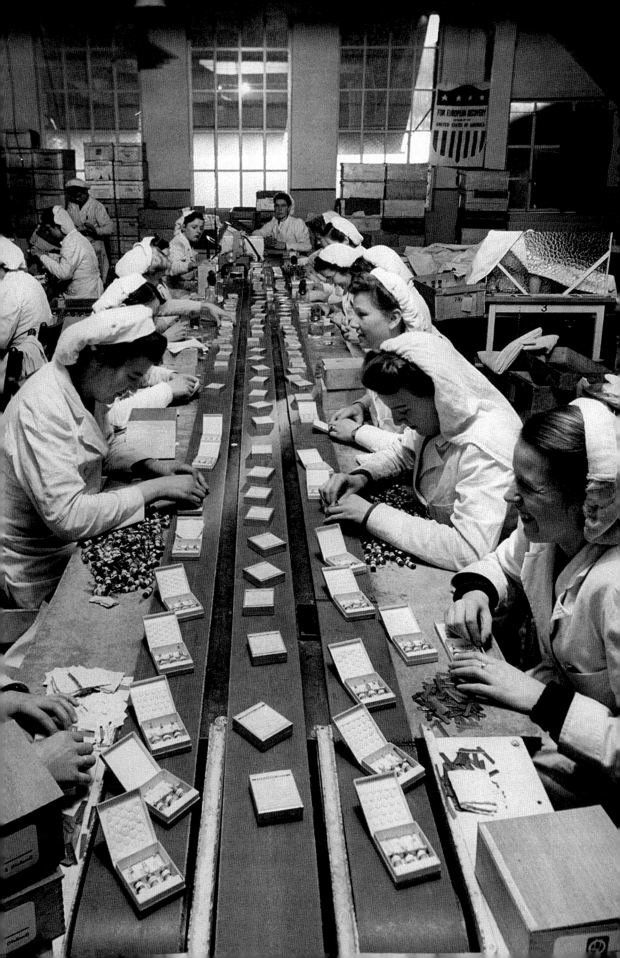

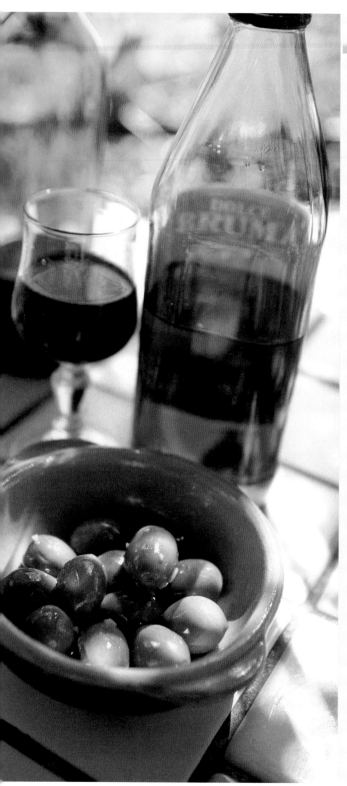

The Mediterranean Diet

What does a Mediterranean diet consist of? Fresh fruit and vegetables reign supreme in Mediterranean countries. Most of the traditional dishes of this region are vegetarian and are generally prepared using fresh ingredients (not frozen). Mediterranean peoples also eat a good deal of fish, some poultry, and almost no beef, pork, or lamb.

The reason for this is that in the Mediterranean climate fruits and vegetables can grow all year round and are relatively inexpensive, unlike in northern Europe and Canada. Naturally, a Mediterranean diet will cost more in winter in these countries.

This diet encourages the generous use of olive oil as the key source of oleic acid (omega-9), known to reduce cholesterol and decrease the risk of developing some forms of cancer. Note, however, that oleic acid is also found in berries, plums, red grapes and their juice, and kiwi fruit, as well as in apples and apple juice.

Since olive oil is 99 percent fat, moderation is called for, just as for wine. On the other hand, compared to butter, olive oil is definitely much better for your health.

people with Alzheimer's disease. This control group was made up of people with what is called mild cognitive impairment (MCI) and who had just one chance in two of developing Alzheimer's disease in the three-year period following their recruitment.

To assess the preventive potential of the new drugs, researchers assembled two large groups of people with mild cognitive impairment. The participants were given either various protective agents or placebos, and they underwent regular medical follow-up for two to four years after being recruited.

The first family of drugs evaluated belonged to the group of non-steroid anti-inflammatory agents (Figure 41). These drugs are usually used to soothe arthritis pain. As we saw in Chapter 7, in large epidemiological studies done in the mid-1990s, researchers had discovered that people who took this type of drug saw their risk of getting Alzheimer's disease reduced significantly, compared with older people who did not take these anti-inflammatory drugs. Similarly,

studies done on identical twins (monozygotes) showed that the twin who did not develop Alzheimer's disease was often subject to frequent bouts of arthritis. Although it was initially thought that arthritis could perhaps protect against Alzheimer's, it quickly became obvious that it was the use of anti-arthritic drugs that was actually responsible for this protective effect.

Given all of these scientific discoveries, it was suggested for the first time that various non-steroid anti-inflammatory agents be studied in people with mild cognitive impairment, with a view to prevention. One of the first molecules tested was Vioxx (rofecoxib), an anti-inflammatory medication that was taken off the market in 2004 because of its significant cardiac side effects. The researchers also examined its main competitor, Bextra (valdecoxib) or Celebrex (celecoxib), which unfortunately did not have any significant beneficial effect in people with mild cognitive impairment. This drug was also the subject of a massive recall by its maker because of major side effects. Lastly, a generic

OMEGA-3 AND OMEGA-6 FATTY ACIDS

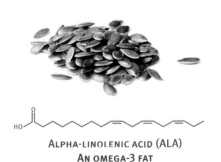

ALPHA-LINOLENIC ACID (ALA)
AN OMEGA-3 FAT

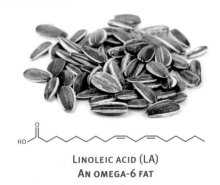

LINOLEIC ACID (LA)
AN OMEGA-6 FAT

FIGURE 40

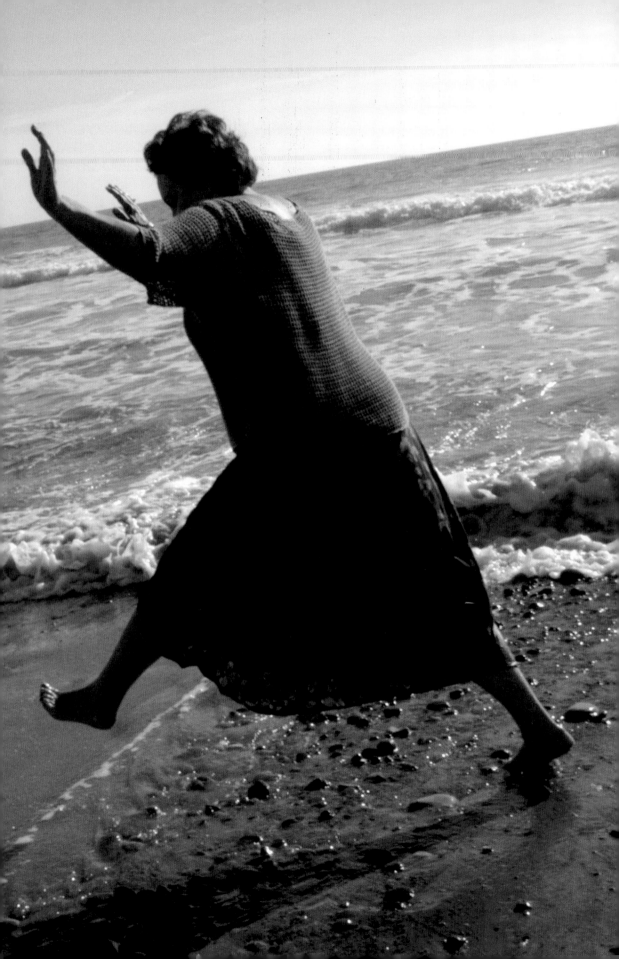

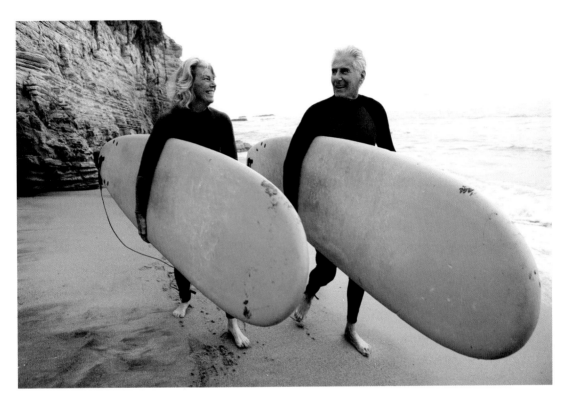

drug from the family of non-steroid anti-inflammatory agents, called naproxen, was studied. The latter study proved to be the most interesting of all, as it rapidly became obvious that the use of this generic drug seemed to cause a significant delay in the onset of Alzheimer's disease in a very specific group of patients: those who were recruited into the study with absolutely no signs of memory deficits. Unfortunately, subjects who exhibited modest memory deficits at the time of recruitment failed to be protected by the drugs after a while.

Several complementary studies are now underway in the United States and Canada to determine the extent to which this particular family of drugs is able to reduce the risk of developing Alzheimer's disease, and whether the effect observed can be replicated in different populations.

We also need to determine why a distinct group of patients seem to have been selectively protected, while other sub-groups of patients who took the same drug still got Alzheimer's disease. Is it a question of particular genetic susceptibility? The presence of other diseases? Other non-genetic risk factors? These fundamental questions will be systematically studied in the coming years.

The second preventive approach studied recently in the United States did not target people with mild cognitive impairment, but instead older people in the general population and who, by virtue of their family history, seem to have a heightened risk of getting Alzheimer's disease. This very expensive American study followed several thousand patients over a period of almost eight years. The drug tested was a concentrated extract of the ginkgo biloba plant, which scientists obtained by enriching the

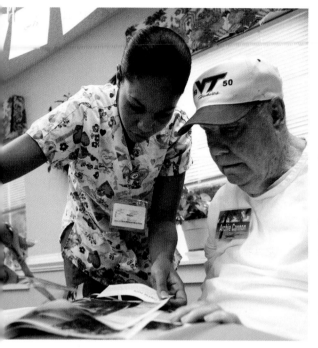

biological fraction of the plant showing the most powerful antioxidant activity.

Doctors administered the ginkgo biloba extract to a group of patients, while at the same time giving a placebo to another group, to determine accurately whether the onset of Alzheimer's disease can be delayed by using a very powerful antioxidant agent. The results presented recently show that this approach has no protective effect whatsoever on people at risk of getting Alzheimer's disease. To this study can be added another done in 2005 on people with mild cognitive impairment, to whom a concentrated dose of Vitamin E was given for three years. Once again, the onset of Alzheimer's disease in people at risk could not be delayed.

MAIN NON-STEROIDAL ANTI-INFLAMMATORY DRUGS

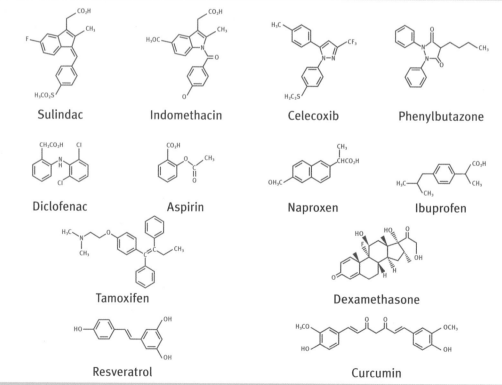

FIGURE 41

Source: *Oncogene* (2004) 23, 9247

That said, recent failures with relatively simple molecules — Vitamin C, Vitamin E, celecoxib (Celebrex) — have nonetheless made it possible to set up the infrastructure necessary to conduct new large-scale studies on prevention in North America and Europe. This research has also enabled scientists to examine and validate several biological markers that will soon be used in conjunction with the analysis of symptoms to better understand and predict when and how a person gets Alzheimer's disease. Lastly, because of this research, the brain imaging methods best suited to monitoring the progression of the disease have been identified, even before the onset of the first symptoms in people at high risk.

In other words, we now know how to go about simultaneously monitoring changes inside the brain and subtle changes in symptoms and memory function, as well as certain biological and genetic changes in people who are transitioning to Alzheimer's disease. It is now clearly established that we will be able, in the relatively near future, to begin to use experimental drugs that are more sophisticated than vitamins and other generic drugs used up to now to slow down and even delay the onset of Alzheimer's disease in people who are genetically predisposed or simply at high risk. Second-generation experimental prototype studies should look something like this:

- First of all, we will determine, in the general population, the people who are at highest risk of developing Alzheimer's disease. These people will have none of the classic symptoms of Alzheimer's disease, but they will have one or two clearly identified genetic risk factors. Brain scans will show that these people have significant neuronal damage or already well-established amyloid deposits, despite the absence of notable symptoms. Once the control group has been identified, the participants will be randomly given either the experimental drug or a placebo. This prototype study will likely last for five to ten years.

- In contrast to drugs currently available on prescription, the experimental drugs being studied will be designed to modify the biology of the brain directly, so as to slow down or stop the degenerative process typical of the disease. In other words, we will no longer just try to reduce symptoms, but will instead try to change the way the disease progresses over time.

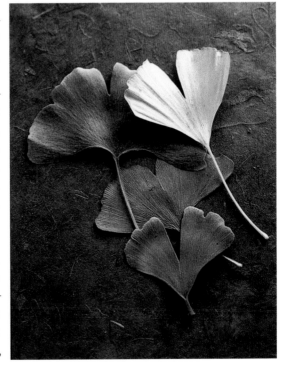

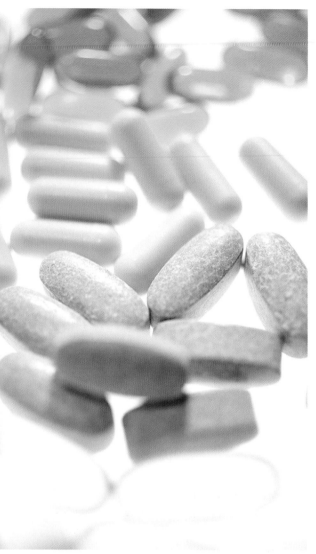

We cannot end this section on prevention without briefly discussing results obtained recently from modifying lifestyle variables.

For example, it has been discovered that people with Alzheimer's disease who adopt a Mediterranean-type diet see a slight slowdown in memory decline; even more important, mortality is reduced significantly. The specific biological mechanisms at work in this phenomenon are still somewhat unclear, but the phenomenon seems to be very real. Furthermore, studies carried out in the United States between 1992 and 2006 in healthy older people have shown that a Mediterranean-type diet combined with regular physical exercise can reduce the risk of onset of Alzheimer's disease by more than 35 percent, compared with healthy people who do little or no exercise and eat an ordinary diet.

Conceivably, therefore, having people at risk, but symptom-free, consume this kind of well-planned diet, may have even more positive effects on the occurrence of Alzheimer's disease, and still more so if a serious regular exercise program is added.

In this vein, we should also mention a recent very interesting Swedish study that examined the positive effects of a diet enriched with omega-3 and -6 fatty acids (from animal and plant sources) in people with Alzheimer's disease, but with varying genetic predispositions. The results of the study are very surprising, but on the whole logical. Only those people with the lazy APOE4 gene, which we discussed at length in previous chapters, saw any (slight) improvement in their situation from taking omega-3 and -6, while people who did not have this defective gene did not reap any benefit from taking fatty acids.

The most promising avenues of research today involve either non steroid anti-inflammatory drugs or pharmacological agents that modulate defective genes, like the lazy apolipoprotein E gene.

These approaches will obviously teach us a great deal about the disease and its progression in the phases preceding the onset of the first symptoms. With sustained research, we will succeed in stopping this twenty-first century scourge in a few years' time.

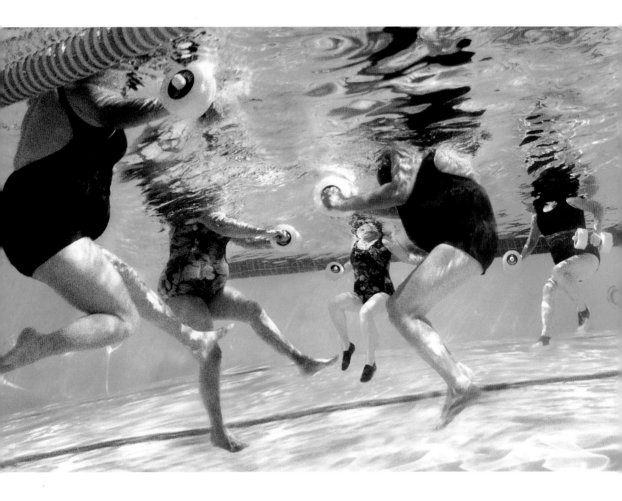

This new science, called pharmacogenetics, involves closely examining an individual's genetic profile before administering a drug. This has enabled us in recent years to understand why some drugs work very well in one person and not at all in another. The reason is that the kinds of genes we inherit from our parents have a huge influence on the action of drugs and the intensity of certain side effects such as nausea and vomiting.

This emerging science has taken giant steps in a short time. Most experimental drugs now being studied are being tested in patients whose overall genetic profile has first been accurately established.

We are slowly moving toward a kind of "individualized" medicine, in which patients will of course be given the treatment best suited for their disease, but adapted according to the nature and behaviour of the genes passed on by their parents. Pharmacogenetics will enable us to move away from the current approach, based on trial and error, and better target appropriate treatments.

Today, we can no longer ignore the scientifically demonstrated benefits that changing lifestyle habits offer and their impact on the risk of developing Alzheimer's disease. We have every right to expect, in the coming decades, to be able to measure

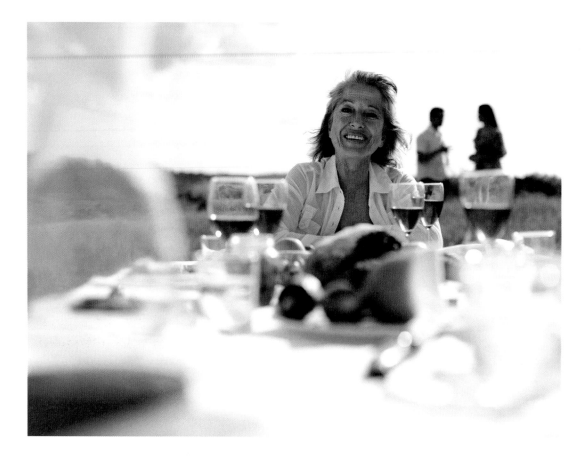

concretely the benefits of better control of cardiovascular factors:

- Elevated cholesterol levels
- Diabetes
- High blood pressure
- Metabolic syndrome
- Obesity

Given that the use of drugs to reduce cardiovascular risk is becoming common worldwide, and is no longer the exclusive right of the western world, we can expect an indirect but significant reduction in the incidence and prevalence of Alzheimer's disease.

Currently, the extent of these benefits is extremely difficult to measure, given the creation of several generic drugs used to control risk factors. However, in the next thirty years these drugs will certainly have a much greater influence on the risk of getting the disease than they have had in the last twenty years.

In Summary

The Shape of Things to Come, or
Medical Research in the Years Ahead

Therapeutic research no longer simply aims to lessen the symptoms of the disease, but rather to stop its progression and even prevent its onset. The control of risk factors like cholesterol, diabetes, high blood pressure, and inflammation with drugs offers promising pathways to solutions. Attempts are being made, as well, to directly target the defective genes associated with the disease, such as amyloids and apolipoprotein E. Recent discoveries suggest that these treatments must be individualized, since each person has distinct genetic baggage and tends to react differently to prescribed medications.

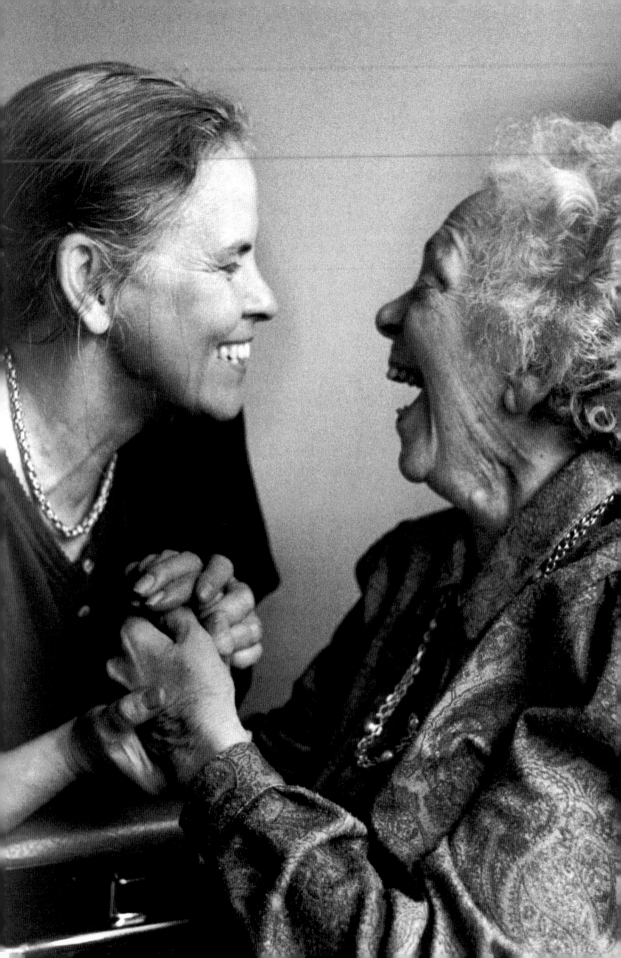

CHAPTER 9

The Major Decisions to Be Made Over the Course of Alzheimer's Disease

A number of decisions have to be made by anyone diagnosed with Alzheimer's disease and by their loved ones. Some are simple, others, agonizing. We think it is useful to talk about these decisions here, in the order in which they arise. This prior knowledge will make it easier to manage care in the various stages of the disease.

THE FIRST VISIT TO THE DOCTOR

Many people with Alzheimer's are not aware they are having difficulties in their day-to-day lives. For example, they have to be reminded about their hairdresser or doctor appointments, birthdays, or expected visits. Their bills are paid late or not at all. They may have forgotten where they parked their car on the street or have lost their wallet somewhere in the house, which often makes them suspect

theft. When their family tells them there has been a change and they need a medical exam, they often reply that "there is no problem." When the family insists, they may change the subject or even get angry. This "anosognosia," or non-recognition of the disease, reduces their own anxiety somewhat, but not that of those close to them!

Other people recognize immediately that they are showing symptoms, especially with regard to memory, and want to consult an expert. Ideally, even in the very first stage of Alzheimer's disease, a person should be accompanied by someone close when he or she goes to see the family doctor. This consultation "on memory problems" may coincide with an annual visit to the physician or involve a separate visit, but more than one visit will certainly be necessary to take the person's history and conduct the appropriate examination.

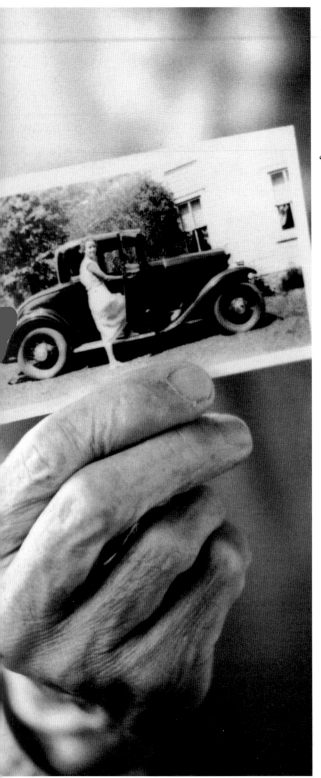

What advice can we give to families when a person showing symptoms refuses to go to the doctor? Sometimes you have to make an appointment "for both of us at the same time," or pretend to go together "for a vaccination." Talking about Alzheimer's disease is not compulsory at this stage; it is simpler to call it "an annual memory exam." However, it is useful to tell the doctor ahead of time so he can better plan the visit.

The first visit is generally to the family doctor. People with no family doctor as such, which is often the case, can visit a walk-in clinic. The person or the accompanying individual can, however, require the doctor on call to arrange a consultation in one of the many memory clinics located in Canada, in the United States, and in France.

After the diagnosis, care is often managed jointly by the clinic and the family doctor, whose office is usually located closer to the affected person's home.

ONCE THE DIAGNOSIS IS CONFIRMED, DOES THE PERSON HAVE TO BE TOLD?

The general rule is to tell to a person with Alzheimer's disease the truth if he or she asks a direct question — "Doctor, do I have Alzheimer's disease?" — unless there is a risk of a catastrophic reaction, that is to say, a reaction involving depression or intense anxiety causing a great deal of distress and perhaps even leading to a suicide attempt. This is relatively rare, considering the large number of people who go through this experience. Normally, the doctor, with the help of those close to the patient, assesses this risk before revealing the diag-

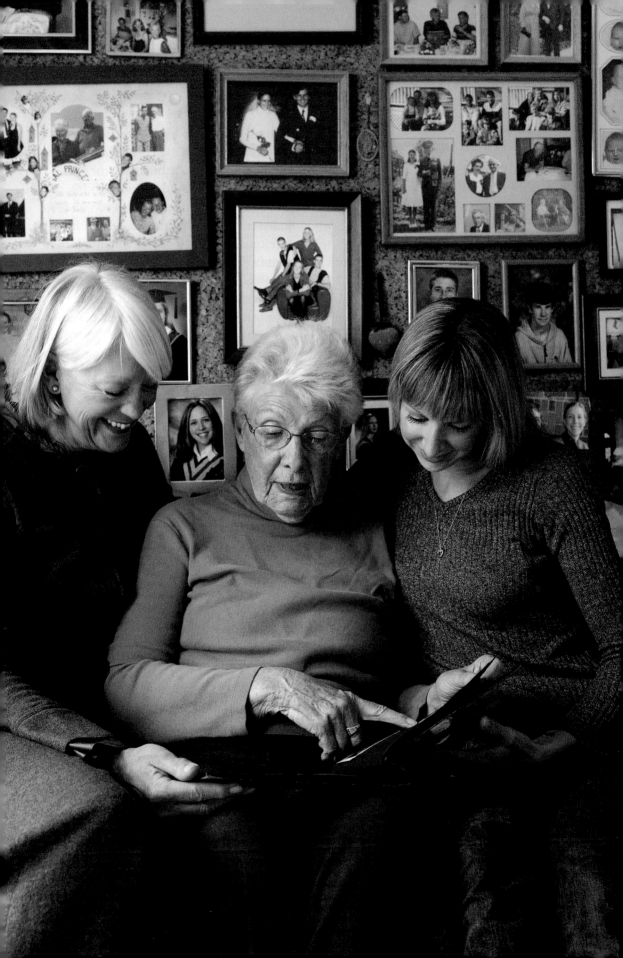

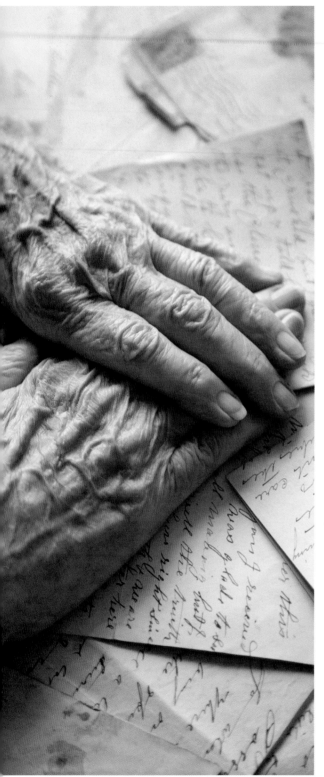

nosis to the affected person. In scientific literature this is known as progressive disclosure, or giving information gradually depending on the questions asked by the person with Alzheimer's disease.

On the other hand, the doctor must inform a proxy or a trusted person as soon as the diagnosis is confirmed, since a series of critical issues will have to be dealt with in the short term, and decisions will have to be made regarding, for example, a health-care proxy in case of incapacity and power of attorney, the ability to drive safely, safety at home, financial management, and many other subjects.

A HEALTH-CARE PROXY IN CASE OF INCAPACITY AND POWER OF ATTORNEY

It is increasingly common for an adult to choose a proxy (called a "substitute decision-maker" in Canada) in advance, in the event a disease or accident renders the individual unable to make informed choices independently at a later date. Given the disease's inevitable stages, a person with the disease absolutely must make this choice while he or she remains competent and in full possession of his or her faculties. The document most recommended is a combination of a power of attorney and a health-care proxy in case of incapacity, prepared in the presence of a lawyer in Canada. The usual clauses are:

- The transfer of financial decisions to a close relative or friend, named as substitute decision-maker — in other words, the person henceforth entrusts the administration of personal finances to a third party.

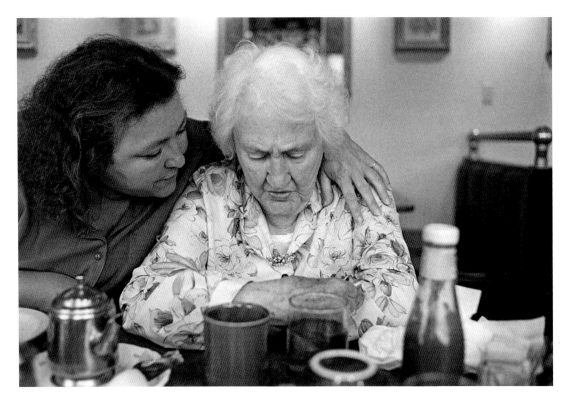

- The transfer of medical decisions to a close relative or friend, named as substitute decision-maker–in other words, the person entrusts future medical decisions to a third party.

This document may also contain clauses that clearly define the intentions of the person with the disease:

- Consent (or not) for cardiac resuscitation — does the person want attempts made to resuscitate him or her following cardiac arrest, a stroke, or other trauma, or not.
- Consent to artificial life support (or not).
- Interest in participating in medical research — that is, trials of experimental drugs or other diagnostic or therapeutic interventions.

Usually, the spouse and at least one child, a brother or sister, is chosen to be the substitute decision-maker. If this document is not done early enough and the person becomes mentally unfit, the family must see a lawyer to make the appropriate arrangements, which vary from province to province.

Following a diagnosis of Alzheimer's disease, it also becomes very difficult to make or change a will, as any change could be contested after death by a frustrated heir. An expert opinion on competence can always be given by a medical specialist before the will is executed, but experience shows that the will is nearly always annulled when it was drawn up after the diagnosis was confirmed, if it is contested with the support of a second opinion. This kind of approach thus results in extra costs with very little chance of success.

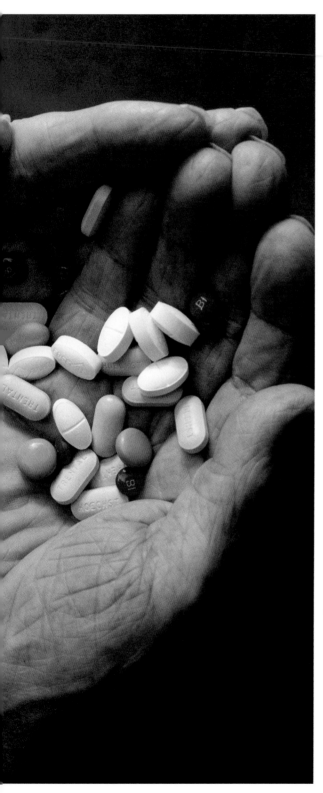

To avoid any ambiguity, futile expenditures, and frustration, it is better to plan ahead: it is essential to hire a lawyer to prepare both a will and a health-care proxy in case of incapacity, documents attesting to the choices and wishes of the individual in question. A clear situation will make the patient's life and that of loved ones easier. The costs are not prohibitive and the benefits will be enormous.

DOES THE PERSON HAVE TO TAKE DRUGS FOR ALZHEIMER'S DISEASE?

Currently available drugs are not cures, but they reduce some symptoms in more than half of people for a year or two. The most recent data suggest that a combination of the two groups of drugs that act on acetylcholine and glutamate significantly delay admission to a long-term care facility; in effect they keep people in the mild to moderate stages longer. It is common in medical practice to try at least one or two of these drugs for a minimum period of six months and then to assess the effects, which vary greatly from one person to another. Fortunately, side effects are weak and reversible.

We should add that easily treatable diseases, such as depression and some vitamin deficiencies, like B12, may accompany Alzheimer's disease. It is often necessary to treat these problems before reaching a final diagnosis of Alzheimer's disease.

CAN THE PERSON STILL DRIVE A CAR?

Let's be realistic: Everyone with Alzheimer's disease will have to stop driving at some point. Depending on the province of residence, the law allows for a degree of flexibility and a driver's licence can be gradually modified by limiting a person's driving to small cities or familiar small towns, or requiring the driver to be accompanied by another adult. A road test administered by the driver's licence office or by an occupational therapist attached to a hospital or expert clinic may be required. If close family members and friends are concerned about the ability of a person with Alzheimer's disease to drive, the attending physician must be told right away; he or she can request the suspension of a licence through official channels. Note that having a driver's licence withdrawn is generally less of a problem for women than men; men sometimes have a tendency to resist having this privilege taken away from them and, in some extreme cases, may decide to drive without a valid licence. In a situation like this, the family or spouse will have to intervene (with something like "the car has broken down!").

The ideal is to encourage people to make the decision on their own, since many patients well understand the impact of the disease's symptoms on the ability to drive a vehicle. A gradual decrease in allowable driving distances makes the transition to not driving at all easier. The worst solution, but sometimes the only one, is to get rid of the vehicle.

CAN THE PERSON LIVE ALONE AND STILL BE SAFE?

Many women with Alzheimer's disease live alone for a period of time, causing worry for the family. There may be danger signs: food in the refrigerator that is long past its

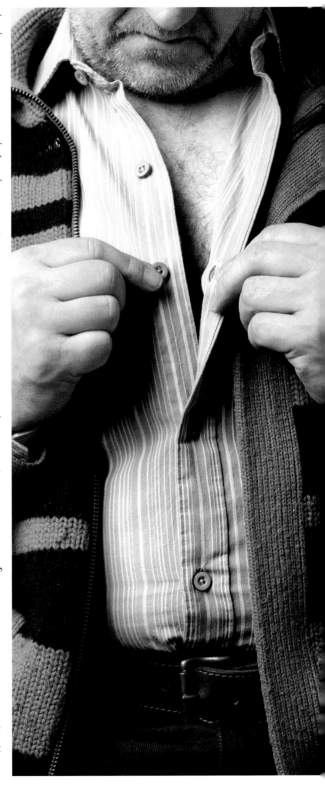

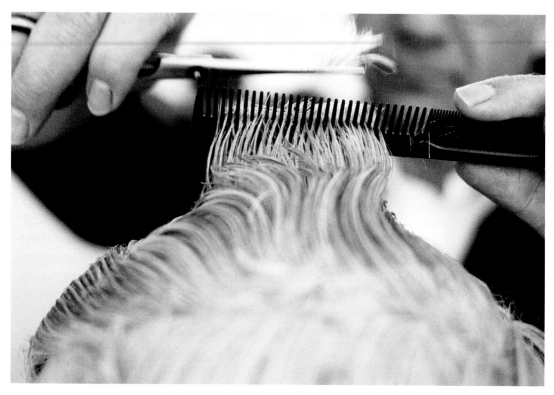

sell-by date, an unlocked front door, a stove or kettle left on and unwatched, invitations to strangers to come into the house. Cigarettes may also become a problem with time, mainly because of the fire hazard. At the request of the attending physician, regular home visits by a third party may help reassure everybody: a female social worker, an occupational therapist, or a government services nurse. This involves home care service programs in the Canada. Medication can be managed jointly by the home care services and the pharmacist who prepares the medication for each week in a box (individual packs) or a blister pack (Dispil). Meals on wheels can be asked to come by once or twice a week to deliver complete meals.

Home help is available once a week. Wearing an emergency medical alert bracelet such as those made by LifelineTM,

which gives a person the ability to activate an alarm or contact medical emergency services long-distance, is strongly recommended for people living alone and who are at risk of falling.

These services are offered at a reasonable monthly cost and the family can ask the organization providing the services to communicate regularly with the person living alone to make sure everything is fine.

Loss of autonomy must be prepared for with the help of a local community health centre. It is possible to visit "service-providing residences." In this kind of facility, a range of services are offered individually according to the person's needs: the administration of medication during the day at the appropriate times, meals in a common dining room, laundry and housekeeping, twenty-four-hours-a-day emergency service, bus transportation to a shopping centre, excursions, etc. Usually, a nurse is always on site during the day and a general practitioner makes weekly visits. In Canada, most services that help the elderly remain self-sufficient are partially reimbursed by the various levels of government, in the form of tax credits or pension supplements.

CAN THE PERSON GO OUT ALONE?

In Canada's northern climate, tragedies occur in winter when people go outside, get lost, and die of cold. Too often these are people with Alzheimer's disease who have escaped the notice of those around them. There is a fairly simple explanation for this phenomenon. As the disease progresses, not only do memories disappear, so do spatial landmarks.

In practical terms, imagine that a person, when leaving his house, has no difficulty recognizing his neighbour's fence, the front of the house across the street, the fire hydrant on the corner, the traffic light across from the restaurant, etc. But on the way back, he only remembers how his street looks viewed from his own balcony, with no recollection of the same landmarks seen from the opposite direction! This street, in fact, bears no resemblance whatsoever to what he remembers. Understandably, therefore, he may easily walk right past it. This is where the wandering phenomenon stems from. The person is looking for a group of landmarks that he usually sees in a certain way, from a certain perspective ... but he doesn't find them.

Those looking after people with Alzheimer's disease need to prepare for spatial disorientation by making them wear an identification bracelet provided by the

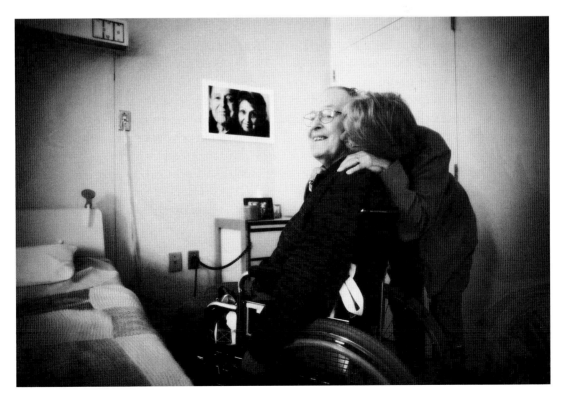

Alzheimer Society of Canada, with a unique identification number that will help police officers bring the lost person home. The possibility of using a GPS to more quickly locate people who are at risk of wandering off, or "running away," is now being discussed.

Sometimes a latch must be installed high enough on doors opening outside to prevent people from going out, since it is not uncommon for people with Alzheimer's disease to get up in the middle of the night because of sleep disorders.

WHAT SHOULD YOU DO IF THE PERSON GETS ANGRY?

Various mood and behaviour disorders may occur at different stages of the disease.

A few details about these disorders should be mentioned:

- These mood and behaviour disorders are not permanent.
- They are often triggered by an external phenomenon (a noise, darkness) that can be modified.
- Sometimes these symptoms will have to be treated with one or more drugs, but only for a limited time (usually no longer than three months).
- Giving the person sleeping pills is not recommended, as they often cause falls and increase nocturnal confusion.
- It is a good idea to consult the attending physician, the Alzheimer's Society, and support groups in nearby com-

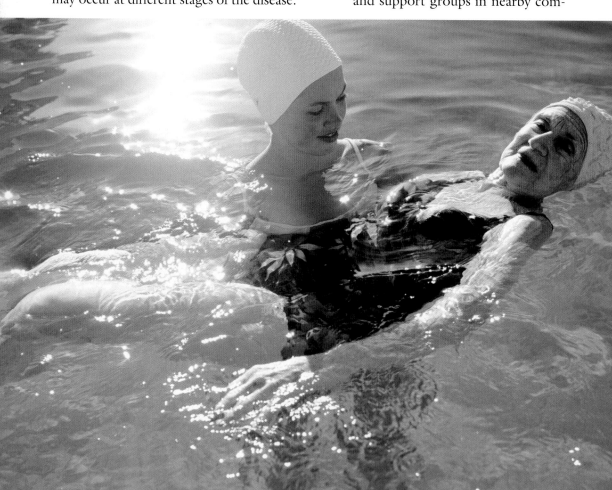

munity health centres to better understand and manage these disorders.

Aggressive behaviour can become a significant source of stress and exhaustion for the informal caregiver or nursing staff. This is often the factor that triggers the issue of placing the person in a care facility: "Is it time?" These behaviours often make providing care more complicated and especially affect quality of life. Fortunately, physical violence, which is quite rare, can be avoided with a little tact: this means not restraining the person or using force, remaining calm and agreeing with what he or she says. This kind of anger is often cyclical and occurs more often toward the end of the day. It is important to determine the source of the frustration and try to lessen the effects.

The temporary use of drugs is sometimes necessary and must be discussed with the attending physician. Luckily, these lapses are usually short-lived, but they will be sufficiently disturbing to get the family to start thinking about the need to plan for long-term institutional care.

WHEN IS IT TIME FOR THE PERSON TO GO INTO A NURSING HOME?

Faced with a situation that is almost inevitable in western societies and cultures, this is probably the most agonizing decision a close relative has to make. In certain obvious circumstances, institutionalization is urgently required: the person lives alone, is badly nourished, or falls frequently. There are intermediate facilities, or "residences with services," small or large, that may be all that is needed for a period of time.

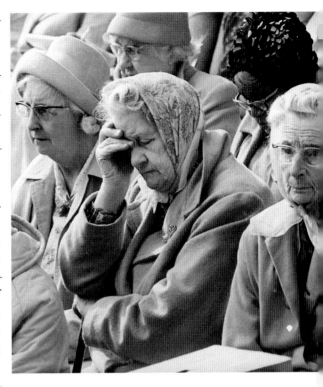

Establishing an active file with your health-care provider quite early in the progression of the disease is recommended, in part to get maximum benefit from home-care services and intermediate resources, but also to plan in the medium term (from six to twelve months) for the need for long-term institutional care. Two forms have to be prepared — a medical evaluation form, the "Classifications according to types in area of long-term care," as well as a form completed by a social worker — which will be sent to a regional allocation authority. This body will decide if the person needs a minimum of daily services and, if this is the case, how urgent it is for him or her to be transferred to a long-term care facility. The family can indicate a preferred facility according to location, and the person's language and cultural group. The wait time ranges from a few months to a few years,

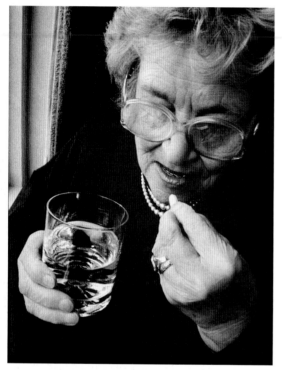

There is no clear decision-making process to tell us the right time to stop administering drugs. Several factors, such as the rate of decline, the patient's general condition, concurrent diseases, and the duration of the disease are taken into account when decisions are made.

SHOULD A CASE OF PNEUMONIA BE TREATED?

Pneumonia is the most frequent cause of death. We often see it coming when people with Alzheimer's disease choke while drinking, and then while eating. It is then customary to ask the proxy (or guardian) what level of appropriate care to provide:

- Transfer the person to a hospital for "resuscitation."
- Keep the person in the current location and treat him or her with oral antibiotics.
- Keep the person in the current location and provide comfort care such as oxygen and morphine via a skin patch.

depending on the location chosen. There are also new specialized private care facilities in which a whole floor is devoted to caring for people with Alzheimer's disease. However, the annual cost of these private or semi-private centres is quite high.

CAN THE PERSON STOP TAKING DRUGS?

Some drugs taken for a long time to prevent a heart attack are no longer needed after a certain age. Other drugs increase confusion, while still others are no longer appropriate for someone who cannot walk or has lost a great deal of weight. Naturally, therefore, the nursing home's doctor and his team will discuss with the proxy (or guardian) the possibility of gradually withdrawing drugs when they are no longer deemed useful.

Making a decision is not usually too difficult if the person's quality of life is taken into account. On the other hand, it will be much easier if the affected person has made sure to express clearly, in a health-care proxy, his or her precise wishes concerning resuscitation, comfort care, and other possible treatments. Often, this discussion will have provided an opportunity to decide whether to undergo autopsy to confirm the exact cause of death and nature of the disease, and whether to preserve the brain in a bank to contribute to medical research into the causes of the disease.

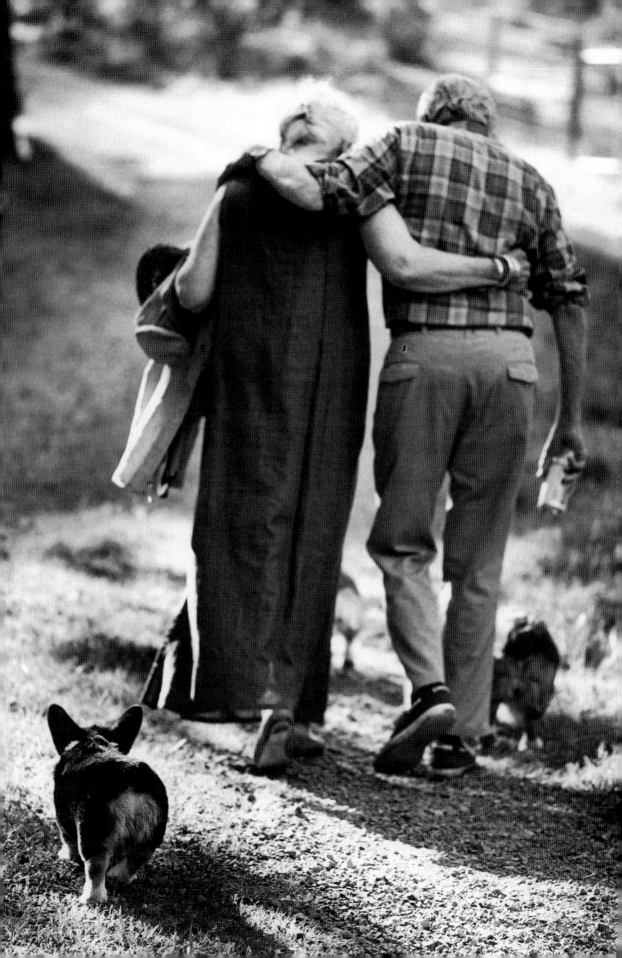

WHEN SHOULD ACTION BE TAKEN TO PROTECT THE HEALTH OF THE CAREGIVER?

Looking after a spouse or a relative with Alzheimer's disease and keeping the person at home is a very significant source of stress, and sometimes calls for great physical effort. Informal caregivers often reach their limits and collapse under the pressure. As we have seen, many important decisions rest on their shoulders over the course of the disease. What's worse, as the disease progresses, caregivers become more and more isolated, to the point where they lose control of their social life. Moments of respite become more and more rare, and adult home day care services such as Baluchon Alzheimer are hard to find both in Canada and in France. It is not uncommon for an informal caregiver's sleep to be extremely disturbed, leading to exhaustion and accumulated fatigue. Discouragement and sadness are common and are too often deemed normal in light of the situation. Be careful! It is precisely at this stage of discouragement that symptoms of depression appear. The most common signs of depression are permanent fatigue, physical pain, and weight loss. Furthermore, depression dulls brain functions, leading to a chronic loss of interest and desire to do anything.

Before reaching this stage, it is crucial to become familiar with the services offered to patients and caregivers. Most local Alzheimer societies host mutual assistance and support meetings for patients and caregivers, and home daycare services are available to allow caregivers to get out and have a break. Family members can also be called on and can share the responsibilities: there is nothing shameful about asking for help! At the first signs of depression, caregivers should consult their doctor to see what can be done. Physical activity is beneficial not only for patients, but also for their caregivers. In short, caregivers have to fight isolation and make use of available services. The worst thing is to do nothing, since both the caregiver and the person affected will suffer as a result.

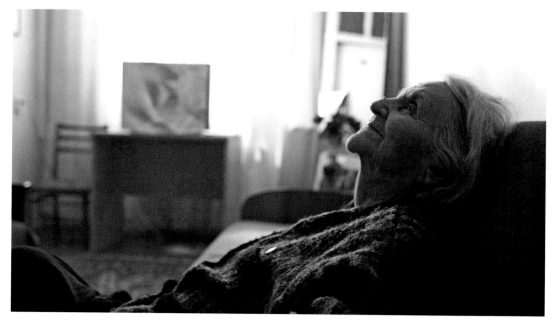

In Summary

The Major Decisions to Be Made Over the Course of Alzheimer's Disease

A person with Alzheimer's disease rarely goes to the doctor of his own volition. It is up to family members to be vigilant and to make the person undergo thorough memory testing so that action can be taken as soon as needed.

The diagnosis must not be hidden from the person affected, but it is best to reveal it in stages, over the course of several visits. A relative or an informal caregiver must therefore be informed about the situation, as a number of decisions will have to be made in the months after the diagnosis.

In conjunction with the person affected, a health-care proxy in case of incapacity must be prepared, as well as a will and a notarized power of attorney, entrusting the management of the person's assets to a third party so that finances are managed appropriately. The issue of driving a car must also be discussed with the attending physician. An administrative procedure is in place for the doctor to inform government authorities of the risk and the need to withdraw a driving licence. The decision to begin procedures to get the patient into full-time care in a specialized institution is the result of a process that usually involves the attending physician, a social worker, and government authorities. Appropriate documents are required.

Ceasing to administer drugs used for treating Alzheimer's disease is a delicate subject. There is no magic formula for determining the right time to do so.

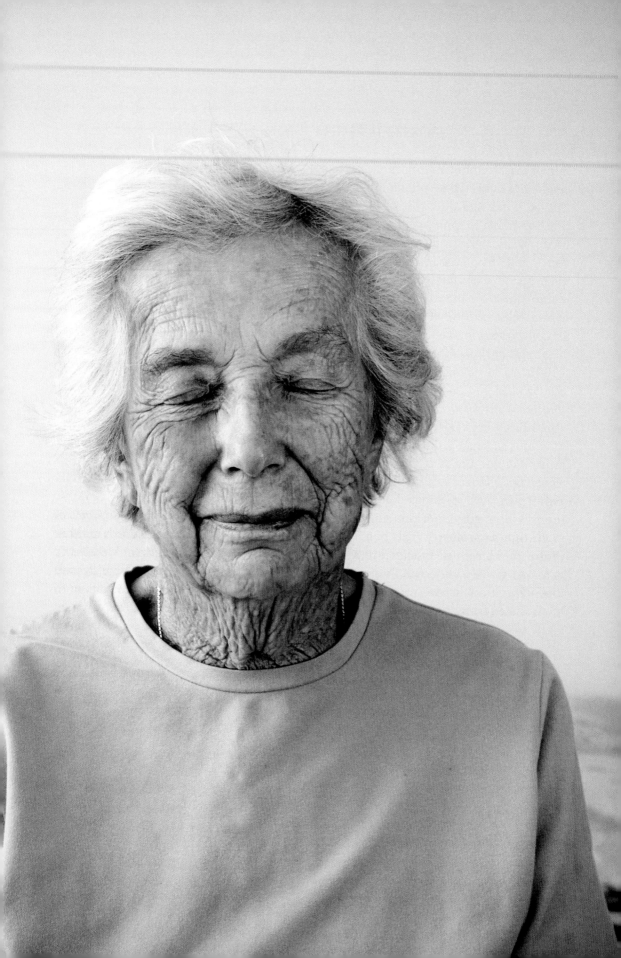

CONCLUSION

A Hundred Years of Progress and Hope

"You already have to have learned many things before knowing how to ask about what you don't know!"

Jean-Jacques Rousseau

We have seen in the various chapters of this book that the medical field has made a tremendous amount of progress since Professor Alzheimer's initial discoveries almost a hundred years ago.

With respect to the so-called "purely familial" forms, we are now aware of three genes that are directly responsible for triggering the disease in a number of families scattered around the world. Systematic efforts are being made to locate these families and encourage them to participate in targeted therapeutic research.

As for the late-onset sporadic form of Alzheimer's disease, we have discovered genetic variants that significantly affect the degree of risk of getting the disease, the age at which the disease begins, and even the rate at which it progresses. These genetic variations will be able to help us choose the best therapeutic approach for each individual, as we are now able to do for some cancers.

Furthermore, four symptomatic drugs (which specifically tackle the symptoms of the disease) were developed by the pharmaceutical industry between 1990 and 2000. A great many therapeutic trials have been conducted or are now underway to find new molecules likely to slow down and even stop Alzheimer's disease. Despite several failures since the approval of the last drug in 2006, we have learned a great deal from these clinical studies and have refined even further our understanding of the disease and the molecular mechanisms that cause brain cells to die.

Over the last decade, from a diagnostic perspective, we have made great strides in our ability to recognize Alzheimer's disease at increasingly earlier stages. For example, in 2004, the demographic data in the Canadian Study of Health and Aging (CSHA), combined with statistics on the sales of drugs used to treat Alzheimer's disease, showed that out of the roughly 250,000 people with Alzheimer's disease at that time, barely 20 percent had been appropriately diagnosed and given suitable treatment. To everyone's surprise, almost 15 percent of people had been given a diagnosis but were taking no medication. Lastly, 65 percent of Canadians with the disease had received neither diagnosis nor treatment.

There were many reasons for the unfortunate situation that existed less than ten years ago. Among the most important were prejudices that die hard even today: memory loss is completely normal after a certain age — even if the case is serious! Or: depression or Alzheimer's, it's all the same thing; it will pass. At the time, we even heard family doctors say they strongly doubted the validity of the scientific studies that led to the approval of drugs now used to treat Alzheimer's disease.

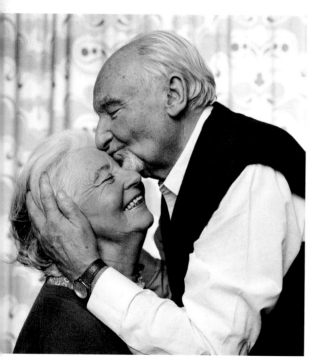

These attitudes can quite easily be explained if we compare Alzheimer's disease with Parkinson's disease. When we administer the first dose of an anti-Parkinson's drug, the improvement with respect to trembling, slowness, and rigidity is obvious in just a few minutes. In the case of Alzheimer's disease, a reduction in symptoms may not be seen for up to three months. Sometimes, the most visible result is the absence of further decline, as compared with a rapid improvement such as that seen in Parkinson's subjects.

Alzheimer's disease is therefore different from various other diseases occurring in elderly people, which means that expectations with regard to response to medication must be brought in line with reality. A patient suffering from diabetes will also experience a reduction in symptoms that is subtle and not easy to see, despite taking medication.

Fortunately, the diagnostic situation has greatly improved since the Canadian data was published in 2004. Since then, the number of subjects diagnosed has skyrocketed, as has the prescription of anti-Alzheimer's drugs. Furthermore, using new diagnostic criteria for detecting Alzheimer's disease that take into account measurements of brain metabolism obtained through tomography scanning, a diagnosis can be made before the stage where the patient is no longer self-sufficient.

Finally, for approximately the past four years the idea of prevention has been in the foreground of medical research in western countries. This situation has arisen to some degree in reaction to the difficulty we are having in developing drugs that are effective in stopping the progression of the disease. There is even a renewed

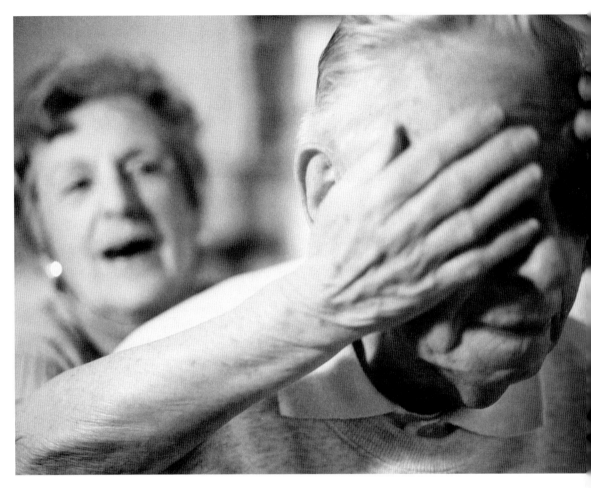

dynamism in university research centres, which have designed and initiated very large-scale studies using vitamins E and C, anti-inflammatory medications, and even ginkgo biloba as preventive treatments. While they have not led to the discovery of a treatment to prevent the disease, these studies have shown governments and the pharmaceutical industry that this ambitious kind of approach can be undertaken while still keeping costs under control. Now that the feasibility of such studies has been established, it is time to move on to the next stage. Specifically, these studies laid the groundwork for a number of well-structured studies now

underway, with the aim of analyzing the benefits of exercise and a Mediterranean-type diet.

New preventive studies are being prepared to assess different types of anti-inflammatory agents as well as certain anti-diabetes and anti-hypertension therapies for people without symptoms. In addition, research into new drugs for people who already have the disease continues to forge ahead and the results of these efforts will be made public in the coming years.

We see this clearly in new trends being reported in the media: older people, as well as baby boomers, who are moving full steam ahead into their retirement years, are making an effort to get more exercise and eat better than preceding generations. It will surprise no one to learn that they are very anxious about brain diseases, especially Alzheimer's disease, since it most often strikes the growing twenty-first century cohort of elderly people. Sophisticated statistical studies now allow us to say this with certainty: if scientists were today able to delay the onset of Alzheimer's disease by just two years, there would be a reduction of more than 26 percent in the number of people affected in less than a generation. Better yet, if we were able to delay the onset of Alzheimer's disease by roughly five or even ten years, there would be 50 to 90 percent fewer people affected.

Seen from this angle, the goal of delaying the onset of Alzheimer's disease appears much more realistic than that of reversing the loss of brain cells, which, as we have long known, has very little chance of success, even if we place our hopes in stem cell technology.

The future thus looks promising, although the scientific and medical challenges remain considerable. Our exhaustive understanding of the disease leads us to foresee new therapeutic solutions we did not suspect even five or so years ago. The proliferation in North America and Europe of new research centres dedicated to the prevention of Alzheimer's disease signals a new phase in medical research on the causes of and treatments for Alzheimer's disease, one full of promise and hope.

Afterword

I am writing these lines just a few weeks after my mother's death, which occurred at dawn on June 2, 2011. But my mourning really began at least fifteen years ago. All these years, I was by her side, to her last breath, in the tragic labyrinth of Alzheimer's disease, which took from her all that she was. Beautiful and eloquent, a fighter for social justice, equity, equality between men and women, the right to education, democracy, freedom. Principles she defended courageously, by taking risks, especially under the reign of terror of François Duvalier and his bloody Macoutes in Haiti. Rebellious, vivacious, passionate about literature and opera, a tireless altruist, but also a loving mother, always worried about her two daughters, whom she had to raise alone when exile led her to cross the ocean and start again from scratch in Canada, in Quebec. She did so while coping with many hardships and worries.

Luce Depestre, my radiant mother and my heroine. She deserved to rest and reminisce about everything she had accomplished and everything she helped us — we, her children, and how many others — accomplish.

I was very close to her and, when the first symptoms of the disease began to take their toll, I desperately tried to understand what was happening to her: Was it depression following a work accident that had forced her to take leave, or an undiagnosed cerebro-vascular disorder, or perhaps the result of circumstances and family tensions that deeply distressed her, or even all of these at once? She could no longer follow a discussion nor participate in it, became more and more silent, was sometimes incoherent, and had panic attacks. Doctors — at least four — and naturopaths she consulted on her own, alarmed to feel herself sinking into a state where everything seemed to be fading away, did nothing other than prescribe a staggering cocktail of sleeping pills, tranquillizers, antidepressants, vitamins, and placebos of all kinds. When I became aware of this, I got angry with the pharmacist who — above all a businessman — had ignored the dangerous overlap of prescriptions without ever questioning the doctors.

My many calls for help to social workers earned me a few disagreeable comments suggesting I was unwilling to accept that my mother was getting older. My worry was all the more justified by the fact that she wasn't even sixty-five!

Then, during an interview with a major specialist on Alzheimer's disease, none other than Dr. Serge Gauthier, I understood, as I listened to his replies to my questions, that the symptoms he was describing corresponded in a disturbing way to what I had noticed in my mother's more and more puzzling behaviours. "Will you let me give her some tests?" he asked me when I told him after the program about my distress. The diagnosis was confirmed — and it was like a dagger in my heart!

For years, the journey was painful and exhausting. I became an "informal caregiver," in other words, my mother's mother. In addition to my weighty professional, personal, and parental responsibilities, I had to look after everything for her: outstanding bills, significant amounts of money she was cheated out of, care, hygiene, shopping, anxiety attacks, delirium, confusion, denial, and rebellion. As a psychiatric and geriatric nurse, she knew what lay ahead. For months, I had to prod social services to get emergency home help, which they could not offer more than two or three hours a week. Then I had the nightmarish experience of very expensive private services and of allegedly supervised apartments for old people who were losing their ability to be self-sufficient, very attractive at first sight but where quackery, dangerous incompetence, and abuse, for want of rigorous government monitoring, are widespread. Finally giving up, for her own protection — as her case was getting worse and worse and I was just about exhausted — I was able to get her placed in extremis on a long waiting list for a nursing home. I have to say that making the decision to place someone in a care facility, almost considered to be a crime in my native culture, was agonizing.

My whole-hearted gratitude goes to the teams of the Alzheimer Society, to the public health nursing and medical staff, who were respectful of the patient's dignity, attentive, devoted, and skilled. They helped me find the respite and calm needed to better help my mother and maintain contact with her, even when she became completely bedridden, and speech, memory, and all her cognitive faculties had left her, right through to palliative care. Mum, through you, with you, by your side, I've grown up.

In this remarkable and very useful book, I have read again everything I learned when I interviewed Dr. Gauthier and even more about the size of the challenges that Alzheimer's disease poses for us, individually and collectively. The recurrence of this disease in my family gives me reason to worry about the genetic factor. Investing in research, protecting the sick, helping loved ones — all are of fundamental importance.

The Right Honourable Michaëlle Jean
27th Governor General and Commander-in-Chief of Canada (2005–2010)
Special Envoy to Haiti for UNESCO

For Further Reading

Chapter 1: Professor Alois Alzheimer: A Scientist with Heart

Engstrom, E. J. "Researching dementia in imperial Germany: Alois Alzheimer and the economies of psychiatric practice." *Culture, Medicine and Psychiatry* 31, no. 3 (2007): 405–12.

Goedert, M. and B. Ghetti. "Alois Alzheimer: His life and times." *Brain Pathology* 17, no. 1 (2007): 57–62.

Maurer, K., S. Volk and H. Gerbaldo. "Auguste D. and Alzheimer's disease." *The Lancet* 349, no. 9064 (1997): 1546–49.

Verhey, F.R. "Alois Alzheimer (1864–1915)." *Journal of Neurology* 256, no. 3 (2009): 502–03.

Chapter 2: A Disease of Epidemic Proportions

Alzheimer's Disease International. *World Alzheimer Report 2010, The Global Economic Impact of Dementia*. London: Alzheimer Disease International, 2010.

Gauthier, S., ed. *Clinical Diagnosis and Management of Alzheimer's Disease*. Oxford (UK): Informa Healthcare, 2007.

Wilmoth, J.R. "Demography of longevity: Past, present and future trends." *Journal of Experimental Gerontology* 35, nos. 9-10 (2007): 1111–29.

Chapter 3: Diagnosing Alzheimer's Disease

Cummings, J.L., M. Mega et al. "The neuropsychiatric inventory: Comprehensive assessment of psychopathology in dementia." *Neurology* 44, no. 12 (1994): 2308–14.

Dubois, B., H.H. Feldman et al. "Research criteria for the diagnosis of Alzheimer's disease: Revising the NINCDS-ADRDA criteria." *The Lancet Neurology* 6, no. 8 (2007): 734–46.

Gélinas, I., L. Gauthier, M. McIntyre and S. Gauthier. "Development of a functional measure for persons with Alzheimer's disease: The disability assessment of dementia." *American Journal of Occupational Therapy* 53, no. 5 (1999): 471–81.

MCKHANN, G., D. DRACHMAN et al. "Clinical diagnosis of Alzheimer's disease: Report of the NINCDS-ADRDA Work Group under the auspices of the Department of Health and Human Services Task Force on Alzheimer's Disease." *Neurology* 34, no. 7 (1974): 939–44.

MCKHANN, G.M., D.S. KNOPMAN et al. "The diagnosis of dementia due to Alzheimer's disease: Recommendations from the National Institute on Aging-Alzheimer's Association workgroups on diagnostic guidelines for Alzheimer's disease." *Alzheimer's & Dementia* 7 (2011): 263–69.

NASREDDINE, Z.S., N.A. PHILLIPS et al. "The Montreal Cognitive Assessment, MoCA: A brief screening tool for mild cognitive impairment." *Journal of the American Geriatrics Society* 53 (2005): 695–99.

POULIN DE COURVAL, L., I. GÉLINAS et al. "Reliability and validity of the Safety Assessment Scale for people with dementia living at home." *Canadian Journal of Occupational Therapy* 73, no. 2 (2006): 67–75 (available at www.sepec.ca/grillesecu.htm).

CHAPTER 4: The Natural Progression of Alzheimer's Disease

DUBOIS, B., H.H. FELDMAN et al. "Research criteria for the diagnosis of Alzheimer's disease: Revising the NINCDSADRDA criteria. " *The Lancet Neurology* 6, no. 8 (2007): 734–46.

DUBOIS, B., H.H. FELDMAN et al. "Revising the definition of Alzheimer's disease: A new lexicon." *The Lancet Neurology* 9, no. 11 (2010): 1118–27.

MAYEUX, R., C. REITZ et al. "Operationalizing diagnostic criteria for Alzheimer's disease and other age-related cognitive impairment, Part 1." *Alzheimer's & Dementia* 7 (2011): 15–34.

REISBERG, B., S. H. FERRIS, R. ANAND et al. « Functional staging of dementia of the Alzheimer type." *Annals of the New York Academy of Sciences* 435, no. 1 (1984): 481–83.

CHAPTER 5: Current Treatments for Alzheimer's Disease

BELLEVILLE, S., F. CLÉMENT et al. "Training-related brain plasticity in subjects at risk of developing Alzheimer's disease." *Brain*, doi:10.1093/brain/awr037. Published on-line March 22, 2011.

BELLEVILLE, S., F. CLEMENT et al. "Training-related brain plasticity in subjects at risk of developing Alzheimer's disease." *Brain* 134 (2011): 1623–34.

DEKOSKY, S.T., J.D. WILLIAMSON et al. "Ginkgo biloba for prevention of dementia: A randomized controlled trial." *Journal of the American Medical Association* 300 (2008): 2253–62.

FORETTE, F., M.L. SEUX et al. "The prevention of dementia with antihypertensive treatment: New evidence from the Systolic Hypertension in Europe (Syst-Eur) study." *Archives of Internal Medicine* 162 (2002): 2046–52.

GAUTHIER, S., B. REISBERG et al. "Mild cognitive impairment." *The Lancet* 367, no. 9518 (2006): 1262–70.

KIVIPELTO, M., T. NGANDU et al. "Risk score for the prediction of dementia risk in 20 years among middle aged people: A longitudinal, population-based study." *Lancet Neurology* 5, no. 9 (2006): 735–41.

VELLAS, B. AND P.S. AISEN. "Early Alzheimer's trials: New developments." *The Journal of Nutrition, Health & Aging* 14 (2010): 293.

CHAPTER 6: One Hundred Years of Research into the Possible Causes of Alzheimer's Disease

DOBLE, A. "Excitatory amino acid receptors and neurodegeneration." *Therapie* 50, no. 4 (1995): 319–37.

GATZ, M., C.A. REYNOLDS et al. "Role of genes and environments for explaining

Alzheimer disease." *Archives of General Psychiatry* 63, no. 2 (2006): 168–74.

GOEDERT, M. AND M. G. SPILLANTINI. "A century of Alzheimer's disease." *Science* 314, no. 5800 (2006): 777–81.

LAMBERT, J.C., S. HEATH et al. "Genome-wide association study identifies variants at *CLU* and *CR1* associated with Alzheimer's disease." *Nature Genetics* 41, no. 10 (2009): 1094–99.

LEDUC, V., S. JASMIN-BÉLANGER AND J. POIRIER. "APOE and cholesterol homeostasis in Alzheimer's disease." *Trends in Molecular Medicine* 16, no. 10 (2010): 469–77.

LINDENBAUM, S. "Understanding kuru: The contribution of anthropology and Medicine." *Philosophical Transactions of the Royal Society B: Biological Sciences* 363, no. 1510 (2008): 3715–20.

POIRIER, J., J. DAVIGNON et al. « Apolipoprotein E polymorphism and Alzheimer's Disease." *The Lancet* 342, no. 8873 (1993): 697–99.

ST GEORGE-HYSLOP, P.H. "Piecing together Alzheimer's." *Scientific American* 283, no. 6 (2000): 76–83.

CHAPTER 7: Everyday Risk and Protective Factors

AMIEVA, H., H. JACQMIN-GADDA et al. "The 9 year cognitive decline before dementia of the Alzheimer type: A prospective population-based study." *Brain* 128, no. 5 (2005): 1093–1101.

BELLEVILLE, S. "Cognitive training for persons with mild cognitive impairment." *International Psychogeriatrics* 20, no. 1 (2008): 57–66.

BREITNER, J.C. AND M. F. FOLSTEIN. "Familial nature of Alzheimer's disease." *The New England Journal of Medicine* 311, no. 3 (1984): 192.

BREITNER, J.C., B.A. GAU et al. "Inverse association of anti-inflammatory treatments and Alzheimer's disease: Initial results of a co-twin control study." *Neurology* 44, no. 2 (1994): 227–32.

CASTELLANI, R.J., R.K. ROLSTON AND M.A. SMITH. "Alzheimer disease." *Disease-a-Month* 56, no. 9 (2010): 484–546.

FRISARDI, V., F. PANZA et al. "Nutraceutical properties of Mediterranean diet and cognitive decline: Possible underlying mechanisms." *Journal of Alzheimer's Disease* 22, no. 3 (2010): 715–40.

KATZMAN, R. "Education and the prevalence of dementia and Alzheimer's disease." *Neurology* 43, no. 1 (1993): 13–20.

LARSON, E.B., L. WANG et al. "Exercise is associated with reduced risk for incident dementia among persons 65 years of age and older." *Annals of Internal Medicine* 144, no. 2 (2006): 73–81.

WILLIS, S.L., S.L. TENNSTEDT et al. "Long-term effects of cognitive training on everyday functional outcomes in older adults." *Journal of American Medicine Association* 296, no. 23 (2006): 2805–14.

CHAPTER 8: The Shape of Things to Come, or Medical Research in the Years Ahead

AISEN, P.S., S. ANDRIEU et al. "Report of the task force on designing clinical trials in early (predementia) AD." *Neurology* 76 (2011): 280–86.

BALLARD, C., S. GAUTHIER et al. "Alzheimer's disease." *The Lancet* 377 (2011): 1019–31.

DAVIGLUS, M.L., B.L. PLASSMAN et al. "Risk factors and preventive interventions for Alzheimer disease: State of the science." *Archives of Neurology* 100 (2011).

GAUTHIER, S. AND P. SCHELTENS. "Can we do better in developing new drugs for Alzheimer's disease?" *Alzheimer's & Dementia* 5 (2009): 489–91.

KNOPMAN, D.S. "Mediterranean diet and late-life cognitive impairment: a taste of benefit." *Journal of the American Medical Association* 302 (2009): 686–87.

RISNER, M.E., A.M. SAUNDERS et al. "Efficacy of rosiglitazone in a genetically defined population with mild-to-moderate

Alzheimer's disease." *Pharmacogenomics Journal* 6 (2006): 246–54.

CHAPTER 9: The Major Decisions to Be Made Over the Course of Alzheimer's Disease

My mandate in case of incapacity, Les Publications du Quebec, 2011; http://www.curateur.gouv.qc.ca/cura/en/ outils/publications/mon_mandat.html

Wills: Definitions, Government of Quebec; http://www.justice.gouv.qc.ca/english/ publications/generale/testamen-a.htm

Home-care services, Government of Quebec; http://www.msss.gouv.qc.ca/en/sujets/ groupes/seniors.php

Bibliographical and Internet Resources

Books and Documents of Interest in French

Gendron, Marie. *Le Mystère Alzheimer: l'accompagnement, une voie de compassion.* Montreal: Editions de l'Homme, 2008.

Groulx, Bernard and Jacques Beaulieu. *La Maladie d'Alzheimer: de la tête au cœur.* Montreal: Publistar, 2004.

Société Alzheimer du Canada, *Raz-de-marée: Impact de la maladie d'Alzheimer et des affections connexes au Canada*, Toronto, Société Alzheimer du Canada, 2009.

Touchon, Jacques and Florence Portet. *La Maladie d'Alzheimer.* 3rd Edition. Paris: Masson, 2004.

Alzheimer Society of Canada. *Rising Tide: The Impact of Dementia in Canada.* Toronto: Alzheimer Society of Canada, 2009.

Internet Resources in French

Société Alzheimer du Canada (www.alzheimer.ca/french/)

Association France Alzheimer (www.francealzheimer.org/)

Fédération québécoise des sociétés Alzheimer (www.alzheimerquebec.ca)

Baluchon Alzheimer (www.baluchonalzheimer.com)

Alzheimer Belgique (www.alzheimerbelgique.be/)

Alzheimer Montpellier (www.alzheimermontpellier.org/)

Association Alzheimer Suisse (www.alz.ch/f/html/)

Internet Resources in English

Alzheimer Society of Canada (www.alzheimer.ca/english/)

Alzheimer's Association U.S.A. (www.alz.org/)

Alzheimer's Foundation of America (www.alzfdn.org/)

Alzheimer's Disease International (www.alz.co.uk/)

Dementia Guide (www.dementiaguide.com/)

International Dementia Advocacy Network (www.dasninternational.org/)

Alzheimer Europe (www.alzheimer-europe.org/)

Alzheimersdisease.com (www.alzheimersdisease.com/)

About the Authors

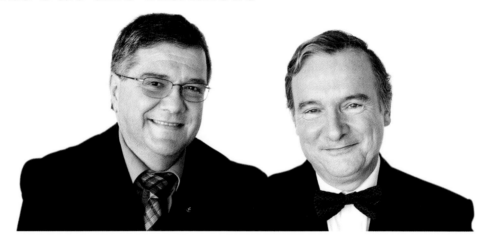

DR. JUDES POIRIER, PHD, C.Q.

Until very recently, Dr. Judes Poirier was director of the Centre for Studies in Aging at McGill University. He is a full professor in the Faculty of Medicine and Department of Psychiatry, and director of the Molecular Neurobiology Unit at the Douglas Mental Health University Institute in Montreal. He is also a career researcher with the Canadian Institutes of Health Research.

Dr. Poirier is a pioneer in biomedical research into the causes and treatments of Alzheimer's and Parkinson's disease. At the Andrus Gerontology Center in Los Angeles he identified the key role of apolipoprotein E (APOE) in repairing brain cells. This major discovery was quickly followed by a second breakthrough that uncovered a genetic variant of APOE that substantially increases the risk of developing the common form of Alzheimer's disease. In 1995 and 1996, he identified a series of genes with genetic variations, making it possible to predict whether certain kinds of drugs will or will not work in a given patient. In some circles he is considered to be one of the founders of pharmacogenomics of the central nervous system.

Dr. Poirier's innovative work has earned him several prestigious awards. Among these are the Beaubien Award from the Alzheimer Society of Canada, the Galien Prize for his contribution in the field of pharmacogenetics, the Jonas Salk Award, and the André-Dupont Prize from Quebec's Clinical Research Club.

In Japan, he was awarded the prestigious International Society for Neurochemistry and First International Parke-Davis awards, for his scientific contributions to the fields of genetics and Alzheimer's disease. He was recently appointed by the premier of Quebec to the rank of Knight of the Order of Quebec. He holds an honorary doctorate from the oldest faculty of medicine in the world, at the Université de Montpellier in France. A scientific ambassador for research related to children (Canadian Medical Research Council) for several years, he is also a businessman and co-founder of two bio-technology companies specializing in pharmacogenomics and pharmaceuticals. One of *La Presse* newspaper's personalities of the week and one of *L'Actualité*'s 1996 personalities of the year, Dr. Poirier is often invited to appear on popular radio and television programs to discuss current developments in research into neurodegenerative diseases, such as Alzheimer's and Parkinson's disease. He is also an international expert on the biology of normal aging and centenarians.

DR. SERGE GAUTHIER, M.D.

Dr. Serge Gauthier studied medicine at the Université de Montréal, did specialty training in neurology at McGill University, and completed a research fellowship in Professor Ted Sourkes' laboratory at the Allen Memorial Institute in Montreal.

He has been a researcher at the Montreal Neurological Hospital, Director of the McGill Centre for Studies in Aging, and Research Chair in the Canadian Institutes for Health Research program for health research and research and development. He is currently a full professor in the Departments of Neurology and Neurosurgery, Psychiatry, and Medicine at McGill University.

His contributions to research include preparing research proposals and conducting random clinical trials to determine the effectiveness and safety of using acetylcholinesterase inhibitors, muscarinic agonists, memantine and molecules capable of slowing the progression of Alzheimer's disease and vascular dementia. Dr. Gauthier has a special interest in a consensual approach to managing dementia in its various stages, in research ethics involving vulnerable people and in the prevention of cognitive losses related to aging.

CONTACT

DR. JUDES POIRIER

Douglas Mental Health University Institute
Perry Pavilion
6875 LaSalle Boulevard
Montreal, Quebec H4H 1R3
Canada

Telephone: (514)761-6131
Fax: (514)888-4094

DR. SERGE GAUTHIER

McGill Centre for Studies in Aging
6825 LaSalle Boulevard
Montreal, Quebec H4H 1R3

Telephone: (514)766-2010
Fax: (514)888-4050

AMÉLIE ROBERGE: 25; 50 b c e f h i; 58; 60; 72; 81 b; 89 b; 90; 92; 110 a

CENTERS FOR DISEASE CONTROL AND PREVENTION: CDC/ Teresa Hammett 81 a

DR. ANNE THESSEN, MARINE BIOLOGICAL LABORATORY, WOODS HOLE, MASSACHUSETTS: 84

DR. SERGE GAUTHIER: 42

DR. PEDRO ROSA-NETO, MCGILL CENTRE FOR STUDIES IN AGING: 46; 49

GETTY IMAGES: Tony Garcia/The Image Bank /Getty Images 12; Peter Adams/The Image Bank /Getty Images 18; Time & Life Pictures/Getty Images 19, 20; Science Picture Co/Getty Images 24; Mitchell Funk/Photographer's Choice/Getty Images 28; Kevin Fitzgerald/Taxi/Getty Images 33; Tino Soriano/ National Geographic/Getty Images 35; Alvis Upitis/ The Image Bank/Getty Images 38, 44; SuperStock/ Getty Images 40; Bromberger Hoover Photography/Workbook Stock/Getty Images 43; Bill Gallery - Doctor Stock/Science Faction/Getty Images 45; Ableimages/Riser/Getty Images 47; Digital Vision/Photodisc/Getty Images 48; Barros & Barros/ Photographer's Choice/Getty Images 51; Hill Street Studios/Blend Images/Getty Images 52; Konrad Wothe/LOOK/Getty Images 54; John Wildgoose/ Photonica/Getty Images 57; Joe McBride/Taxi/Getty Images 60; David Young-Wolff/Stone/Getty Images 68; Robert Decelis Ltd/Photographer's Choice RF/Getty Images 71; ImagesBazaar/Getty Images 73; Piecework Productions/The Image Bank/Getty Images 74; Joe Raedle/Getty Images 76; Laurence Mouton/PhotoAlto Agency RF Collections/Getty Images 78; AFP/Getty Images 80; Genin Andrada/ Cover/Getty Images 82; SSPL/Getty Images 83; Lucille Khornak/Taxi/Getty Images 86; CMSP/Getty Images 87; Steve Satushek/Riser/Getty Images 88; Archive Holdings Inc./Getty Images 89; Chris Knapton/Stockbyte/Getty Images 92; Karen Kasmauski/ Science Faction/Getty Images 93; George Musil/ Visuals Unlimited/Getty Images 95; Andy Sotiriou/ Photodisc/Getty Images 96; Fuse/Getty Images 97, 135; Kevin Laubacher/Taxi/Getty Images 100; Alex Telfer Photography Limited/Photonica/Getty Images 102; Cultura/Nick Daly/StockImage/Getty Images 103; Anne de Haas/Vetta/Getty Images 104, 146; Keystone Features/Hulton Archive/Getty Images 105; Ronnie Kaufman/Iconica/Getty Images 106; Purestock/Getty Images 107; Rubberball/Mike Kemp/Getty Images 108 a; Jed Share/Photonica/ Getty Images 108 b; John Foxx/Stockbyte/Getty Images 109; Chris Everard/Stone/Getty Images 113; Jose Luis Pelaez Inc/Blend Images/Getty Images 116; I. Burgum/P. Boorman/Stone/Getty Images 119; 478697/Getty Images 121; Universal Images Group/Getty Images 122; Steve Gschmeissner/Science Photo Library/Getty Images 124; Sean Justice/ Riser/Getty Images 126; Peter Cade/Iconica/Getty Images 127; MedicImage/Universal Images Group/ Getty Images 128 a; John Still/Photographer's Choice/Getty Images 128 b; Visuals Unlimited, Inc./ Carol & Mike Werner/Getty Images 129 a; Nat Farbman/Time & Life Pictures/Getty Images 131; Bill Boch/FoodPix/Getty Images 132; MCT/Getty Images 136 a; Time & Life Pictures/Getty Images 137; Plush Studios/Riser/Getty Images 138; Altrendo images/Getty Images 140; Sarto/Lund/Stone/ Getty Images 139; Bengt-Goran Carlsson/Nordic Photos/Getty Images 142; Mel Curtis/Photodisc/ Getty Images 144; LWA/Dann Tardif/The Image Bank/Getty Images 145; Bromberger Hoover Photography/Workbook Stock/Getty Images 147; National Geographic/Getty Images 148; Peter Dazeley/ Photographer's Choice/Getty Images 149; Anthony Marsland/Stone/Getty Images 150; JJRD/Vetta/ Getty Images 151; Daniel Day/Iconica/Getty Images 152; R Dumont/Hulton Archive/Getty Images 153; Heather Monahan/Workbook Stock/Getty Images 155; Peter Scholey/Photodisc/Getty Images 154; Hans Neleman/Stone/Getty Images 156; Sam Bloomberg-Rissman/Flickr Select/Getty Images 158; Erik Dreyer/Stone+/Getty Images 160; Steven Puetzer/Photodisc/Getty Images 161

GROUPE LIBREX: 110 b; 118; 120 a b; 125; 129 c; 133 b c; 136 b

LILLY DEUTSCHLAND GMBH: Dr. Konrad Maurer 16

NEW YORK PUBLIC LIBRARY: 21

SARAH SCOTT: 171

SHUTTERSTOCK: Golden Pixels LLC 30; Giorgiomtb 32; Konstantin Sutyagin 41; Carsten Reisinger 50 a d g; Max Blain 58 a; Monkey Business Images 64; Bochkarev Photography 66; matka_Wariatka 75; Michael Drager 111; MaxPhoto 112; Roman Pyshchyk 133 a; Fotohunter 133 b; Elena Ray 134

SPRINGER PRESS, RESEARCH AND PERSPECTIVES IN ALZHEIMER'S DISEASE: Dr. Konrad Maurer 22 b c

THE LANCET: Dr. Konrad Maurer 23

VEER: Alexandr Mitiuc/Veer 26; tepic/Veer 36; Monkey Business Images/Veer 62;Fancy Photography/Veer 98

ZEITSCHRIFT FÜR DIE GESAMTE NEUROLOGIE UND PSYCHIATRIE: Dr. Alois Alzheimer 22 a

Coming in October 2014

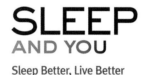

Diane B. Boivin M.D., Ph.D.
Foreword by Ève Van Cauter

Sleep Better, Live Better

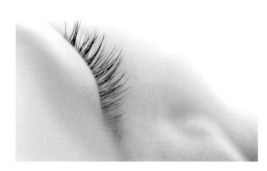

SLEEP AND YOU
Sleep Better, Live Better
By Dr. Diane B. Boivin

Why do we need to sleep? For those of who pass nights staring at the ceiling, the question is beside the point. In fact, we are all sleeping less, and worse, than ever. Despite this, we know that losing sleep or sleeping fitfully has consequences for our health and well being. What can we do when sleep just won't come?

In nine fascinating chapters, Dr. Diane B. Boivin lays out exactly why sleeping well is essential to good health. She explains, in a clear and accessible way, the phenomena associated with sleep: our individual sleep needs; circadian rhythms and problems linked to our biological clocks; the links between insomnia, stress, and obesity; why those suffering from anxiety or depression can have trouble sleeping; snoring; sleep apnea; night terrors; and dreams, among others. Special attention is given to sleep disturbances affecting night workers and new mothers.

An abundantly illustrated, practical guide for everyone trying to reclaim their sleep.

Also from Dundurn

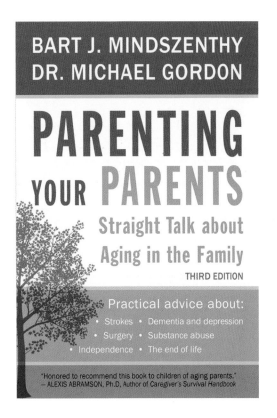

PARENTING YOUR PARENTS
Straight Talk about Aging in the Family
By Bart J. Mindszenthy
Dr. Michael Gordon

Since the last edition in 2006, much has happened in the field of eldercare. There is now an increasing awareness of the complex challenges posed by the expanding aging population in North America. When our parents reach a certain age and have difficulty coping, we find ourselves wondering how to provide them with the kind of love, care, support, and attention they need, just as they have done for us all our lives.

The third edition of *Parenting Your Parents* shows, through twenty-four case studies and the personal experiences of the authors, that you are not alone and offers crucial advice to help you along this difficult but rewarding journey. It also offers a new "Vulnerability Index" to measure what level of need your parents may have right now, as well as a financial planning section and resource directory.

Available at your favourite bookseller

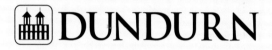

DUNDURN

Visit us at
Dundurn.com
@dundurnpress
Facebook.com/dundurnpress
Pinterest.com/dundurnpress